So many questions!
What a journey!
Oct 20 21
Eleanor

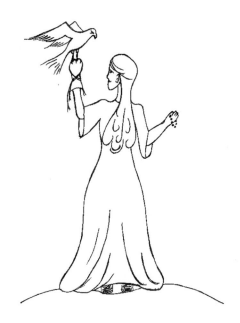

10 Days in April

... a detour through breast cancer

Follow me where I go, what I do and who I know
Make it part of you to be a part of me
Follow me up and down all the way and all around
Take my hand and say you'll follow me.
—*Follow Me, John Denver*[1]

a memoir by
Eleanor Deckert

BOOK 5

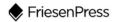
FriesenPress

Suite 300 - 990 Fort St
Victoria, BC, Canada, V8V 3K2
www.friesenpress.com

Disclaimer: This content is not intended to be a substitute for professional medical advice, diagnosis, or treatment. It is a memoir of the author's experiences trying to understand the options and emotions while taking the detour through breast cancer at this time and place.

Author web page: DADEM Studios
Front cover art: Rosalind Gerspatcher
Graphics: Eleanor Deckert
Names of people have been changed to protect privacy.

Seven Predictable Patterns ®

Photos illustrating each chapter can be found on the author's web page
www.eleanordeckert.com

ISBN
978-1-5255-3641-0 (Hardcover)
978-1-5255-3642-7 (Paperback)
978-1-5255-3643-4 (eBook)

1. *Biography & Autobiography, Personal Memoirs*
2. *Family & Relationships, Ethics & Morals*
3. *Self-Help, Green Lifestyle*

Distributed to the trade by The Ingram Book Company

DEDICATION

I dedicate this book to two women I have never met.
They saved my life.

৪০ ✿ ০৪
Rhoda
She died of breast cancer in 1968.
She left her husband and three children:
Lauren age 10
Kathlyn age 8
Matthew age 3
Lauren became my best friend.

I was diagnosed with breast cancer in 2015.
At first, I was confused how this tiny speck of breast cancer
could possibly be life threatening?
Then, I remembered Lauren's Mother.
The reality of the danger prompted me to take action.
৪০ ✿ ০৪

৪০ ✿ ০৪
Louise
That's what I call her. I don't know her real name.
She was my cancer – telephone – buddy.
During my decision-making process and treatment,
she listened to me through every emotion,
shared her story and her faith.
I truly believe I could not have faced these months
without her encouraging, steady, wise, kind words.
৪০ ✿ ০৪

ACKNOWLEDGMENTS

I do not know your names.

You make tea and serve cookies.

You drive the bus and keep the schedule.

You greet people with your smile and fold hospital gowns.

You take turns at the front desk and welcome newcomers.

You run races and collect pledges.

You donate quilts and paintings to cheer the hallways.

You donate money and man the phones.

You are an army of volunteers.

I don't know how you do it,
but I am thankful that you make
the detour through cancer treatments a little easier.

FOREWORD

I hate cancer.

It seems so unnecessary.

— *Lauren (Rhoda's daughter)*

Table of Contents

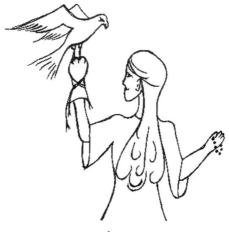

Chapter 1
Wednesday, April 1, 2015
Long Night, Long Day

How long it's been since yesterday.

What about tomorrow?

What about our dreams and all the memories we share?
—*Poems, Prayers and Promises, John Denver*[2]

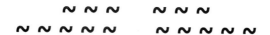

April 1st. A date to remember.

Twenty-eight years ago I was in labour.[3] My husband and Mother encouraged my efforts while Doctor Lam and Nurse Julie attended to my needs. It was my third birth. Doctor Lam had been with me through every delivery. I was experienced and confident and everything went smoothly. If there was time travel I would gladly return to that moment when I first held this darling, warm, soft, precious baby boy in my hungry arms, brought him to my left breast and adored him with my eyes. Stroking his tender cheek, brushing his curls with my fingertips, overflowing with wonder at the miracle of life, I was astonished to see that he was already busy nursing. I was grateful that my body could produce the nourishment he needed. Milk! Life!

Cozy. Safe. The newborn slept. And soon I did, too.

~ ~ ~   ~ ~ ~
~ ~ ~ ~ ~   ~ ~ ~ ~ ~

But, tonight, I don't seem to remember how to sleep.

My husband, sleeping beside me, is so relaxed. I peek at the red numerals on the motel alarm clock. 12:07. I don't think I have slept at all. Cozy memories of life clash with the real hazard of death.

For hours I have been replaying yesterday's events over and over again in my head.

~ ~ ~   ~ ~ ~
~ ~ ~ ~ ~   ~ ~ ~ ~ ~

March 31

"Do you know why you are here?" The slim, young women with the clipboard asked, signalling me to have a seat, her smile attempting to convey a sense of welcome. Her pen was busy filling out some kind of admission form: name, birth date, doctor's name. My husband, Kevin, stood near the door. I gripped the edge of the countertop behind me and remained standing.

"Do I know why I am here?" I feel a volcano inside of me ready to spew fire and brimstone!

"I am here because cancer cells do not die. You have to kill them. Every other cell in the body has a life-cycle and lives, regenerates itself and dies to keep the body in a healthy balance.

Cancer cells only multiply without ever dying. That's why you have to slash, burn and poison them. 'Eradicate.' That is the word my sister-in-law gave me." I stared straight ahead. I did not want to make eye contact with the smiling receptionist in the entry, the smiling volunteers in the hallways, nor the smiling technician interviewing me now.

"I am here because I have already had surgery to remove a tiny speck of breast cancer. However, radiation treatments are intended to kill any rogue cells or undiscovered beginnings. That is why I am here today. The total amount of radiation has been measured out into sixteen treatments. The radiation beams will pass through my left breast on a diagonal to my armpit. Today, it is my understanding, that every new cell that is at the first part of its development, that is in the path of the radiation will be damaged and die. Skin cells, fat cells, nerve cells, hair follicles, sweat glands, mammary glands, milk ducts, blood vessels, muscles, lymph nodes, rib bones, intercostal muscles, lung tissue. It will even skim across my heart. Each of these kinds of cells has a different lifespan. The 'sunburn' that people talk about is because the skin cells live and die and are renewed every fourteen days. So, that is the most noticeable experience of the treatment. But, really, many other cells will also be damaged. I read in one information package that if you feel tingling or sharp twinges, that is the nerve cells growing back even eighteen months after the radiation." I speak in a monotone. I do not dare allow emotion to enter my voice.

"Do I know why I am here? Yes. I am here because no one has figured out how to kill only cancer cells. At the present time, this bulldozer method is what is available. We need an assassin that will go in and take out only the target." That would be a huge break-through!

"I am here because this is what is recommended. I think it is an alarming idea and I am very afraid. I don't want it but I have decided to do it." My hands open and shut repeatedly, gripping the countertop in an attempt to keep myself in the present and prevent my feet from rushing out of the door, down the hallways, out into the open air.

My thoughts are racing. I have no idea how this nasty thing began to grow inside my body! Cancer! I have never smoked tobacco or any other drug. I have never used coffee or alcohol, and avoid food colouring and prepared foods. I have never used any hormonal treatments or birth control pills. I have been growing my own organic food for over 30 years. I breast-fed our four children for more than a year each. I thought breast-feeding almost guaranteed safety from breast cancer! I use herbs to restore the body's natural balance and promote an environment for healing with peppermint tea, ginger, garlic, salt water, yogurt or apple cider vinegar. But this time, changing the environment inside of my body is not enough. I have to kill my own cells in my own body. I am not one bit happy about this. I have never used insecticide or herbicide or spermicide or even mouthwash to kill anything.

Mice and mosquitoes. I have killed them!

"Why am I here? Because my husband is sensible. He told me that babies can have cancer, animals can have cancer, the ancient mummies have evidence of cancer. So, I can see that there is not always a known 'cause and effect' link between lifestyle and cancer." I heave a sigh.

"Yes, I know why I am here. I am here to do something I never ever thought I would have to do. Radiation! I have a very common form of cancer and this is the recommended treatment at this time in history. I am sure someday we will look back at this chapter of medical practice and shudder that this is what so many people have had to endure. I don't want to do it but I have decided to do it." By repeating myself, I hope to feel more brave.

And so, it begins.

The technician looks surprised, writes on her papers, hands me a blue bar-code identity card, opens the door and leads the way. She shows me how to use the card to sign in, where to go each week to get information about my daily appointment schedule, where I will change my clothes, find a hospital gown, and which waiting room to report to.

"Please give this letter to the technicians before my appointment." It is half a page of typing requesting my feeble preferences up against all of this multi-million dollar facility, scientific research and ever-new stream of patients.

Her job is done. I never see her again.

~ ~ ~   ~ ~ ~
~ ~ ~ ~ ~   ~ ~ ~ ~ ~

To the Technicians:
I apologize for my stiff, withdrawn
behaviour, face and interactions.

I do not intend to be rude. I realize you are all doing
fine work. I appreciate the ways you are helpful and
cheerful and have pleasant attitudes and voices.

I am protecting myself. I do not wish to remember this
experience. I do not want to make eye contact,
learn your names, see the equipment, hear
any music, or interact with small talk.

I am very thankful there is a counselling
office where I can communicate.

The city, the machinery, the seriousness of the
word 'cancer' and the isolation I will mostly have
while these days go by is very hard to manage.

So I am going to be on time, to put my things
on the chair, to lie down and cooperate with
your instructions. More importantly, I need to
concentrate on the inner thoughts I am focused
on, and leave as quickly and silently as possible.

I do appreciate your education, voices and efforts.

I am in your room for a few minutes.
I have to take care of myself for the other
twenty-three-and-a-half hours every day.

So, I am letting you know that I am silent on purpose.

Thank-you for the many people you are helping.

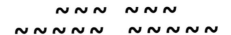

I signed it with my Lifetime Cancer Identification Number.
Because, that is really all I am here. Not a person. A number.

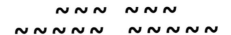

Kevin promised to go in with me. I insisted.
    My name is called.

Through a wide, thick door I see a large room with a flat table in the centre. That's for me. I try not to see anything else. Space-age machinery, metallic gizmos and gadgets, lights, geometric shapes all have no meaning to me. I don't look. I don't want to see. I don't want to remember.

Up on the table, flat on my back, gown open, I follow instructions.

Kevin stands against the wall directly past my feet. I don't look at him, either, but I know he is there, my only, steady, familiar anchor.

"May I hold something in my hand?" I have brought two things with me. As if I was a toddler with a security blanket. As if a good-luck amulet had power to save me. As if I could ride a magic carpet to a safe, beautiful place. As if a sacred object could shield me.

"Yes." There is a smiling face near me that I do not acknowledge.

My right hand clutches a tiny golden eagle pendant and ten purple beads.

There is an arm rest for my left arm up, over my head. My arm is held out of the way so that the radiation will not pass through it. A cross of two straight green lines of light intersect on the tiny ink dot on my sternum. A second tiny ink dot under my arm is the other information needed to get me into the right position. The table is raised and lowered until it is just right. "Move a little to your left." Now my body is oriented exactly for the radiation beam to accurately pass through the targeted area: my left breast.

My left breast, where I first offered life supporting milk to each of our four children. My left breast, which never did anyone any harm. My left breast, which is now the bulls-eye.

I can never undo this. I am saying, "Good-bye." Grief.

And then the two technicians leave the room, signalling Kevin to follow them.

"I'm going now. I'll be just outside the door." My husband's voice is my last link to reality. My last link to my past. It feels like it is the last moment of the 'Back-to-the-Land' lifestyle we have had as our top priority since we got married 37 years ago. It feels like time travel. I am about to fast-forward from my domestic routines in our log cabin, chopping kindling, digging in an organic garden, experimenting with Do-it-Yourself projects, a life of straightforward simplicity to now enter an unknown, futuristic, science-fiction thriller.

The heavy, silent door swings shut. This is the first. I start the count-down. I must repeat this sequence fifteen more times.

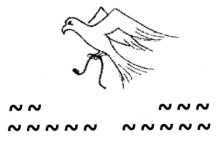

A click. I think the machine above me, to my right, has turned on. A humming. I count the seconds. Another click. I think it is off. Now there is movement. The machine I don't want to look at is moving up and over me, stopping near my lower left. A click. A humming. I count the seconds. Another click.

I feel absolutely nothing.

How can something so powerful result in no physical sensations?

The door opens and I am free to move.

I dress. Walk beside Kevin down the hallways. I don't look at him. I don't look at the pretty quilts and paintings on the walls, donated by artists, intended to cheer the place up. I don't greet the smiling volunteers with their tea and cookies. I just want to make it through the glass doors to the world of Nature, walk on the earth, squint in the sunshine, open my senses to the living plants, become soothed by the rhythm of the rippling lake, notice the sounds of birds, and breathe the open air.

Kevin guides me back to where the truck is parked.

"I can't go yet," is all I manage to say.

∿∿ ∿∿∿
∿∿∿∿∿ ∿∿∿∿∿

We stayed there for two hours.

I had to repeat out loud every bit of information, worry, facts, turning points I had experienced in the past six months. Kevin listened. Calm. Adding sensible comments. Somehow he stayed with me while I wept and wrestled, shouted in whispers, tense and fierce, dizzy and doubt-filled, bewildered and yet, somehow: brave.

"I was so afraid of the radiation, Kevin. All I could think of was the atom bombs, the devastation of entire cities, the screaming, the fires, the scorched earth where no plants or animals live. I was so afraid when I heard the word 'cancer' come out of my doctor's mouth and realized she was talking about me. All I could think of was a day back in the 1960s when a boy in Grade 4 said, 'My mother has cancer,' and we all knew that what he meant was, 'My mother is going to die.' I was so afraid to 'trust the system.' All I could think of was, 'They want my money' as if cancer is a big business and there's actually a conspiracy because they want more customers!" I paused to look out at the peaceful lake, the bobbing daffodils, the children playing in the park.

"Kevin! We chose this 'Back-to-Nature' lifestyle 37 years ago! 'Back-to-Basics!' 'Self-Sufficiency!' We have avoided pollution, rejected man-made chemicals in our environment, avoided processed foods. I have been baking our bread, nursing our babies, weeding the garden, preparing two big freezers full of food we grew ourselves. I have avoided everything unhealthy I have ever heard of and chosen healthy habits at every turn. How can it be that I have cancer?" My voice sounds like wailing. My heart is pounding. "I thought you had to 'do' something to get it. I thought you could 'not do' something and avoid it! What is happening?" The world is a tricky place. Thin ice. Landslide. Monsters lurk. Pounce. Slash.

"Mammograms are such unpleasant things..."

"But, they save lives," Kevin quite rightly interrupts with logic.

"Hospitals are so scary..."

"But, we live in Canada and everything is paid for," again, sensible.

"How do I know the doctor is making good decisions..."

"He has dedicated his time and energy to study this. He wants to do good with his efforts, just like I am careful at my work and you excel at what you do." Kevin's view is helping me see more clearly.

"I hate being a number..."

"But that number entitles you to the benefits of medical treatments." Good point. "And keeps all of your records in one file. You wouldn't want to start all over again." Another good point.

"I want to be my very own, individual, one-of-a-kind drop of water, not melt into the vast immeasurable ocean of cancer patients," somehow my individual identity really matters to me.

Kevin reaches to stroke my hair, touch my hand, turn my face to meet his eyes. "You are. You are my One and Only. I know this is hard for you to do this. But, it is a gift you are giving to me. I don't want to say 'good-bye' to you anytime soon."

Arriving at this huge facility, finding space in this sprawling parking lot, walking through the hallways, sitting in the waiting room, observing staff, it dawns on me how enormous this 'cancer' thing is. And this is just one place, in a fairly small city, in a country with an overarching medical system that everyone can access. My mind zooms out to try to imagine the armies of cancer patients, medical staff, research scientists, lab technicians, and family members impacted by these nasty cells. Today. Yesterday. Tomorrow. Who, when, what will stop this parade?

There's more I have to say. "When you go to the clinic or hospital, there are a variety of people with a variety of problems. Each one has hope that their doctor will suggest an intervention, cure, or procedure to make the problem go away. Here, every single person we see had one diagnosis, 'Cancer.' And they all know people who have died. It's terrifying."

"And they all know people who have survived." It is amazing to me that Kevin can find a positive way to look at things.

"It's strange to see so many people wearing daffodil lapel pins, the symbol of cancer awareness month. My favourite flower! Everywhere blooming! April!" The contrast between the beautiful and the horrible is yet another off-balance sensation to try to manage.

"A symbol of renewal, of hope," Kevin reassures me.

His optimistic efforts are beginning to orient me to be able to hold a more level-headed mind-set.

"One thing I recently realized." My tone of voice has softened, become more thoughtful. "Science has conquered many of the diseases that we used to die from. Diphtheria, scarlet fever, whooping cough, smallpox, polio. Vaccines have prevented childhood deaths." I am named after my grandmother's first child who died at age four from diphtheria.

"And safety equipment, regulations and training have prevented accidents that used to take adult lives," Kevin adds from his experience working with machinery.

"Florence Nightingale taught people to wash their hands. That was a little over one hundred years ago," I think back, fitting scraps of history into a whole. "Understanding microscopic organisms and improving sanitation prevented deaths so cholera, and other contagious diseases were greatly reduced."

I look out again at the families enjoying the lakeside playground. "So many ways we used to die have been almost eliminated. We keep saying, 'Why can't they find a cure?' But, really, now only these degenerative conditions like heart disease, diabetes, muscle and nerve conditions and cancer are left. So far it is not clearly understood how they can be cured or prevented." I sigh and realize, "I guess this is just where we are and what we know at this time and place in history."

Kevin has been following his own line of thinking. "If fame and power and money and worldwide research looking for the best scientific or wildest alternative treatments worked, it would make world news. If there was a 'Magic Bullet' that could save people from cancer, then celebrities and millionaires would take it. But, they get cancer the same as anyone else."

"So what you're saying is that at this moment in time, there really is nothing else for a person to search for. There is no 'Magic Bullet' and all of this 'maybe this' and 'maybe that' is just a wild goose chase?" Well, I feel less hyper now, less anxious that I should be reading scientific data, and doing on-line research, and asking a zillion questions, and doubting every authority figure.

"Kevin, there's one more thing, something kind of fragile to try to put into words," I am so thankful that he has been able to stay with me so patiently through this reorganization of my thoughts. "Some people say, 'Why did God let this happen to me?' I don't feel that way. I have trusted God my whole life and nothing changes that now. But, what I don't trust now, is my own body! How did this happen? What could I have done or not done to have avoided this?" The world feels dangerous with an unexpected ambush or quicksand or pitfalls to trip me up with no warning.

"Michael explained that it's part of the aging process," Kevin remembers the telephone conversations with our son who is involved with cancer research. "Each cell copies itself again and again through our lifespan. People used to have a shorter lifespan, so cancer didn't show up as often. Now, we live longer and when the cells reproduce, an error or distortion in the genes sneaks in and is passed on, multiplying and taking over an organ."

"I still don't get it. Why do you die from breast cancer? My breast has served its purpose. It made a lot of milk. It has no function now. It's not my brain or heart or lungs. How could any sickness in this unimportant body part eventually cause death?" I feel kind of stupid. Maybe other people know the answer to this question, but I don't.

"Cancer builds its own blood supply, taking more and more resources, starving the body." Kevin simplifies the complexity.

"Like a parasite," I get that. "That kills its host." A sombre thought. But, one I can understand.

I have regained my composure now. We sit silently for a few moments. There is much to consider. I feel like spinning puzzle pieces in my head have fit into place and I can see a clearer picture, not the tumbling jumble I started out with.

"I think I understand my mind!" Clarity at last!

"Well, that's a good thing!" he sounds relieved.

"I am *not* just my body," which sounds astonishing by itself. "I am my *story!*"

We have been married for a long time. Kevin recognizes my sudden, creative flash, waits curiously for the rest of my statement.

"I am my decisions. I am my attitude. I am my reaction to things outside myself. My body is a container, a vehicle, a vessel I live in. I act and speak with my body, but the ideas and decisions are the source. I have known people with disabilities, or crutches, or even a person who is dying who is still a real person. Their body is failing, but their 'Self' is still strong." I feel energized and confident. "I cannot prevent what has happened inside my body. But, I do have some say over my reaction, and the decisions I make, and actions I take, and words I say. These come from 'Me.' These make my 'Story.' I am my story!"

For a moment, I experience a calm sense of satisfaction.

"Where's my Journal? I want to write this down!"

Boldly, I step out of the truck, walk on the fresh grass, under the bowing willow trees, near the sandy shore, kissed by the wide, clean water, sitting at a picnic table, Kevin is near me while I jot down my 'A-ha!'

"Look!"

A splendid bald eagle, wings spread wide, is spiralling above us.

"It is just like my eagle necklace! Just like my Falcon!"

~~ ~~~
~~~~~ ~~~~~

It is 2:00 in the morning, April 1.

I may be able to get to sleep for a few hours? Going over the sequence of that first unsettling day, storing up the sweetness of the wise words of my husband, I find a focal point, like an oasis, when I recall the gliding eagle. I allow my mind to travel into the scene I have created to deliberately focus on each time I lie on the bare metal table to receive each of the sixteen treatments.

My fantasy is my shield and shelter from hurricane force emotions and disorienting fears.

~ ~ ~ ~ ~
~ ~ ~ ~ ~ ~ ~ ~ ~ ~

High in the mountains, a rushing snow-fed creek slows across a wide, grassy meadow. Dammed by generations of beavers, the marsh has become a haven for water fowl and nesting shore birds. While the smaller forest folk scamper in the lush undergrowth, this place is also a safe, year-round water source for deer, elk, caribou and both canine and feline hunters. The marsh plants are ideal food for moose. An entire ecosystem of thriving populations interacts here as the seasons cycle. Bears hibernate and bring their young in the spring, feast all summer, return to their nearby den. All is well.

Recently, an observant hiker noticed and reported a sterility in the landscape and lack of animal sign. Naturalists came to determine the cause of declining animal populations and try to understand the imbalance that caused the withered plant life. It was discovered that an invasive breed of eels has been multiplying undetected until the colony now gives off enough waste matter to sour the water and damage the life-cycle of the native plants. Without clean water, without nourishing plants, all other species have no stability here.

A local falconer has been called in. For sixteen days, she will send her trained falcon to hunt the eels. Her left arm is raised, high over her head. She stands tall, fearless, confident in the skill and loyalty of her trusted companion.

After the adult eels are removed, a substance will be dissolved in the water to destroy any eel eggs that are still present. No one knows for sure. Will this method permanently eradicate the poisonous eels?

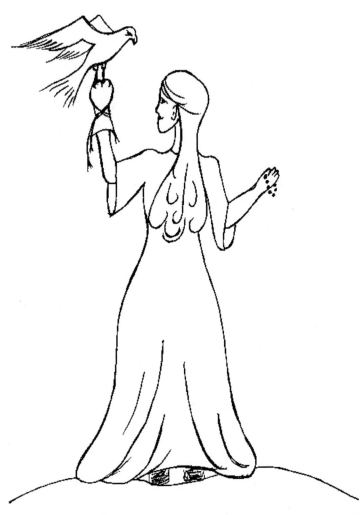

I am the Falconer, with my left arm up-over my head while I lie on the table. The dangerous, slithering, invasive, overpopulated, poisonous breed of eels are the cancer cells, which threaten my internal environment. My Falcon is the radiation beam, power-ful, hunting, destroying. Later, like the water with the dissolved substance to rid the marsh of toxic, undetected eel eggs, my entire body will be safe when my daily medication will prevent any lurking cells from repopulating.

I am confident in my Falcon's skill. I must be silent, motionless and patient while the mighty bird does her work. Soaring and diving, she passes from right to left. Swooping and diving she returns from left to right. Diagonally she cuts the sky and skims the surface of the beautiful life-supporting marsh. I eagerly watch as my Falcon snatches the deadly eels with her deadly talons, removes the contamination, and returns to my care.

New generations of many living things will benefit from this effort.

Every muscle is relaxed. Every thought is calm. Sleep, at last, envelopes me.

~~ ~~~
~~~~~ ~~~~~

5:00 Dawn.

Having my arm up above my head reminds me of something. I can't quite picture it. Some famous person, or scene, or historic moment?

I can see it in my mind. A man, on top of a hill, holding his arms up above his head. Who is that beside him? What is in the valley below him? Why is it so important for him to continue to hold this uncomfortable posture?

I know who it is!

I slide out of bed, open the laptop computer, try to remember Kevin's instructions to go on-line.

"It's someplace in Exodus, I think." I type 'Moses' into the search bar. "Hmm, way too many verses. How about 'Aaron,' his brother?" Still too many possibilities. "There was another man." Two helpers held up Moses' arms. "What was his name?" I close my eyes. I can see the Sunday School picture I coloured as a child.

After the Red Sea. Before the Promised Land. Not Moses with the Ten Commandments. It was a story about a battle. God told Moses that as long as he kept his arms up, the People would win the battle. But, if he lowered his arms, the enemy would win. All day Aaron held up one side and ... who held up the other?

"Hur!"

I found it.

Whenever Moses held up his hand,
Israel prevailed;
and whenever he lowered his hand,
Ameleck prevailed...
Aaron and Hur held up his arms, one on one side,
the other on the other side;
so his hands were steady
until the going down of the sun.
Exodus 17:8–13

Kevin knows a lot about the history of war. Weapons. Machinery. Leaders. Spies. Maps. Dates. Communication. Turning points.

But, when I watch a wartime movie, I follow the family, romance, costumes, music, interpersonal drama. I have never given much thought to the strategies or responsibilities of those in command.

Now I am the commander.

Moses' example guides me. God told him to go into battle. God knew and told Moses how to win. Moses knew, "Some of my own men will be killed. But, in the end, we will prevail... if I do my part."

It has never occurred to me that a general knows he will kill some of his own soldiers.

I have never killed anything in my own body: tobacco, alcohol, cut, burn, pierce, tattoo, mouthwash, spermicide, IUD, abortion. I only gargle with salt water to change the environment, not kill anything.

But, now. It is necessary to kill some healthy cells in order to destroy the deadly cells.

Like Moses, I will hold my arm up during the battle and, with the help of God, in the end, declare a victory.

I have one more Bible verse to search for on-line.

Whatsoever things are true,
whatsoever things are honest,
just, pure, lovely, of good report
if there be any virtue
and if there be any praise
think on these things.
Those things you have both learned
and received and heard and seen me do
and the God of Peace will be with you.
Philippians 4:8

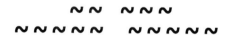

10:00
Radiation appointment Number Two.

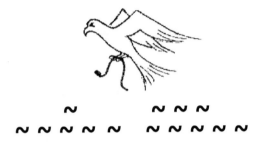

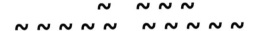

I am so glad that Kevin can come, and see, and wait for me again. I am not doing this for me. I am doing this for him.

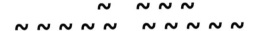

11:00
Kevin and I are waiting in a small meeting room for a consultation appointment I requested with the department head. I try to stay focused on my notes. I don't want to get distracted. I don't want to sound dizzy. I don't want to backtrack and repeat myself. I don't want to waste her time.

I do have important reasons to consult with her.

She will know me by the number they gave me. A seven digit number. Yes, of course, I already have lots of ID in the form of numbers: telephone, address, birth date, social security, credit card, bank account. But I willingly signed up for most of them, and I can change them when I want to. But this? This 'Lifetime Cancer Identification Number' I actually have to keep and refer to it so that all of my records are together and (Dear Lord, Protect me) any future cancer diagnosis and treatments can be recorded. Horrible. Necessary. It feels like a heavy omen hovering there.

It is an open file, ready to collect more data. Just in case. No matter how much I attempt a 'positive attitude' and hope for a satisfactory outcome, there is this dark, ominous question. Will I ever need this number reactivated?

There are, after all, any number of other ways to die! I don't have to believe that cancer will again rear its ugly head, popping up unexpectedly in the same or other breast, bone, lung, liver or brain, perhaps undetected until 'too late' when eventually no treatments will be effective. Maybe I'll die in an accident, or fire, or water, or heart attack, or choke. Maybe I'll never need this 'Lifetime Cancer Identification Number' and will not shrivel, waste away, die and in the end become another statistic.

This number is *not* my 'Lifetime Identity'!

There's no point going over my anxiety. I'm so tired of hearing that the answer to every cancer question is 'maybe.' Do we know how cancer starts? Do we know how to stop it? Do we know how to prevent it? Will this treatment be effective?

'Maybe.'

Michael told me, "You have the most common form of breast cancer and this is the preferred treatment. Are there guarantees? No. From now on, it's a numbers game. Percentages of this. Percentages of that. No one can foresee the future, only measure what has happened so far. From there, you make your decisions."

My first impression of Ms. Department Head is that she is tall, blond, slim, businesslike, perhaps guarded. She handles complaints every day. She makes decisions quickly, firmly. She looks efficient and functional.

Introductions are made.

"My husband and I have been living a rural, do-it-yourself lifestyle. We built our own house. We grow our own food. This is a very foreign environment for me to be in." I let her know where I am coming from. "I have done my best to prepare, educate myself, understand and be ready to cooperate with the procedures here. I like facts. My informed intellect reduces the alarm, which can suddenly flood my emotions." I want her to know that I have made an effort. I'm not here to complain. I do not intend to have an emotional outburst.

"However," I continue, "the literature I read about radiation," I place a stack of officially published pamphlets on the table between us, "seems to blur facts, soften the language, leave room for confusion." I lean forward, opening to sticky notes I marked. "For example, using the word, 'sunburn.' This is a 'nice' word, which identifies something that almost everyone has experienced, but it masks the fact that the treatments impact not only the surface of the skin. The same damage is being done right through the treated area. In another place, when discussing restorative surgery after mastectomy, there was mention that reconstruction was unlikely if radiation had already occurred. I asked my surgeon about this and he said, 'The blood supply is not sufficient to allow for proper healing.' That tells me something I need to know about my own body, but it was not stated. Here is another place. A 'tingling sensation' can be felt eighteen months after radiation because the nerve endings are returning. That means that the nerves were damaged. It is more scary to have this information disguised than for it to be straightforward. It seems unfair to me to use words that are not saying what is really happening."

It is impossible for me to read her carefully inexpressive face.

"Here is another phrase. 'Take your picture.' Does that mean a camera, or an x-ray? I want to know."

I look down at my notes. Gather my thoughts.

"I'd also like to tell you about two major misunderstandings that nearly made me decide not to participate in these treatments.

"Firstly, Dr. O said the radiation would pass through my heart. I thought he meant that it would shine straight down on me, through my whole chest! I was terrified! Later, I found a diagram on-line and I saw that it was a diagonal beam, barely interfering with the organs within the ribs." Now it is hard for me to control my face.

"Secondly, I was told that each appointment would be for 20 minutes. Does that mean that the radiation beam will be on for 20 minutes for 16 times? Do the math! That is terrifying! Later, I learned that it would be on for seconds during each session. A much smaller total." I can't help it. My nerves betray me. My jaw quivers. My voice is shaking. "I'm trying to pay attention. I need facts. 'Don't worry' and 'You'll be fine' are not comments that help me. They only make me distrust the speaker. Dr. O said these platitudes to me when I asked for information."

"You don't seem ready. I don't know if you have given your consent. You've already had one treatment?" She looks at my file.

"No. Two."

"I cannot take the radiation out, you know." Now she makes eye contact with me.

I am talking to an iceberg. A wall.

"Asking questions does not mean I have not given consent. It means I want clarification. I want to learn. I have travelled for five hours. I am here. This is my consent." She is so powerful. I am so small.

"I do feel emotional." I try to explain my situation. "Today is my son's birthday. It is the anniversary of life-giving milk generously produced to supply this precious infant. It is very hard to deliberately aim a deadly force at the place I first held and nourished my newborn son! It seems impossible that I would choose to destroy the miraculous organ that gave life!" I can't hold back the tears. I know my face is tense, red.

"These questions show that you are not ready, that you don't want to be here," she repeats.

Can she actually expel me? Refuse treatment?

"Because I have tears in my eyes? Because I have feelings?" I feel panicky now. "No. I don't want to be here. But I am here.

My priest wears a breast cancer ribbon. My husband wants me to live. My Naturopath said it is OK to use 'two tool boxes.' Lily said, 'Eradicate!' Fred said, 'Throw everything at it.' These people I trust. Therefore, it must be done. Still it is *very* hard to do this. But, I am."

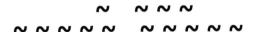

12:00
    Return to motel.
    Eat lunch.
    Nap.

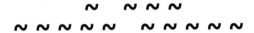

4:00
    How can we celebrate the birthday of our son, Nicholas, today?
    E-mail messages.
    Ice-cream.
    Kevin invites me to the movies!
    What a beautiful retelling of Cinderella!
    Such an excellent way to rest my mind.
    Smile? Did I just smile?

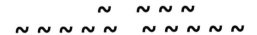

10:00
    I brought CDs of soothing music.
    Eventually, I sleep.
    April 1st. A date to remember.

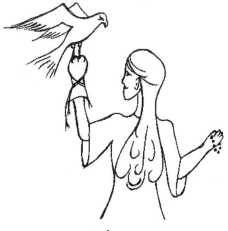

Chapter 2
Thursday, April 2, 2015
The Conveyor Belt

I'll be there when you're feeling down
to kiss away the tears that you cry.
—*For Baby, John Denver*[4]

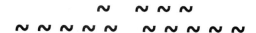

I went in for a checkup with Dr. A in September, which led to a mammogram in October.

The mammogram led to the biopsy with Dr. B in December. Those test results were a cancer diagnosis on January 2nd. Happy New Year! I was immediately referred to Dr. C, a surgeon, who explained vocabulary I had never heard before. The surgery date was set for late January. There was not much to do except stay on the conveyor belt.

The hospital is a two-and-a-half hour drive from our log cabin in the mountains. Because the check-in time was 7:00 in the morning, my husband and I stayed in a motel the night before. "Let's walk," I suggested. It was one tiny decision I could make for myself. It was pitch dark that January morning as we walked seven blocks, climbed the stairs and got back on the conveyor belt.

I was passed from one technician to another. First to the 'Diagnostic Imaging' department for the room with the mammogram equipment. Stripped to the waist, chilly, flattened, injected with a numbing substance, a probe was inserted to locate the cancer. In my hospital gown, with my steady, reliable husband, I walked to the 'Nuclear Medicine' rooms to wait. Four needles to numb so that four needles of dye could be injected near the centre of the breast. The conveyor belt stopped for an hour to wait for the dye to circulate and indicate the sentinel lymph node. A room full of equipment was the next stop along the line to collect images and map how the dye was moving inside me.

I had to harden my heart when it was time to move away from my husband. It became imperative that I blocked all of my emotions.

My surgery was scheduled for noon. At 2:00, it was time.

Except for the hospital bracelet, all physical clues to my identity had been stripped away. Away from my own home. Away from my own clothing. I even had to take off my wedding ring.

"This is it!" I whispered into my husband's hug.

Onto a gurney. Away from my own husband. I was moved along the conveyor belt. Women in scrubs and hair nets wheeled me through hallways. They know. I don't. Just another work day for them. Life changing for me. Rigid with fear, I was strapped to the surgery table while the women moved in their routine duties.

It seemed that everyone knew what to do to take care of my body. I just had to do as I was told. But I felt like 'I' wasn't even there. No mater how much scientific data had been collected about me, 'I,' my 'Self,' didn't seem to matter at all. Invisible. No one was helping me take care of 'Me.' Heart. Soul. Mind. Body. I can stand and sit and walk and wait and put my body or arm here or there and follow instructions. But, what about my emotions? I am not just a body. I am a person, too.

I recognized Dr. C's voice.

"How long does this surgery take?" I asked.

"About an hour and a half," he answered in the voice I had come to trust. "That's counting the lab test." Dr. C had explained that the patient remains unconscious while the diseased tissue is taken to the lab. A dye around the edges indicates that the margins are clear. After that information is passed back to the surgical ward, the patient is prepared for recovery. Meanwhile, the lymph nodes that were identified on the map are removed. The results of those tests would come later.

I glanced at the clock.

My glasses were removed. Being able to see was the last thing that was taken away.

I spoke to Dr. D, the anesthesiologist. As if I was sending up a flare gun to signal 'here I am' I blurted out, "I am more afraid of you than of the surgeon. I get it that the diseased piece needs to be removed. It's just like cutting away the bruise on a banana or an apple. But you, I am afraid of. Today is the anniversary of the day my Dad died after a mistake was made on the surgery table.[5] I don't want to go to sleep now and not wake up."

Dr. D mumbled reassurances from behind his mask. The tray of instruments was in place. Another needle into my wrist. Sleep became irresistible.

~   ~ ~ ~

~ ~ ~ ~ ~   ~ ~ ~ ~ ~

I became aware that I could hear my husband's voice and forced my eyes open. "I'm so thankful. I'm just so thankful!" I kept repeating. I was alive! "What time is it?" I was so relieved to know that indeed, the surgery had taken one and a half hours. Everything must have gone smoothly.

After the required time had passed in the recovery room, I could dress, stand and Kevin helped me into the taxi to return to the motel. It was dark. That whole day I was on that conveyor belt.

I thought I was done. But, no.

Appointments were set up in sequence through February. Dr. E set up the bone scan. Dr. F supervised the CT scan. Dr. G, my dentist, was updated about my diagnosis and treatment plan. Dr. H took a Pap tissue sample. I wanted to cross every test off the list. I signed up for a colonoscopy with Dr. I. Next, I want a strange lump on my throat to be looked at, so I am sent to the eye, ear, nose and throat Dr. J. She assigns me to an ultrasound. One more thing. What is this patch on my skin? Dr. K takes a look and a biopsy.

Is there any more cancer?

Thankfully: No.

Meanwhile, I decided to contact three homeopathic doctors.

First, I asked Dr. L, "If it was you, would you take radiation treatment?" I was surprised by his answer.

"Yes," he said, referring to the cancer cells, "You have to kill the little bastards."

I spent most of my appointment with Dr. M, the second homeopathic doctor, in tears. He reassured me that it was good to think of both methods of medical treatment as two tool boxes. The standard medicine and the natural medicine could complement each other.

The third, Dr. N, suggested I have my blood work done to test for vitamin D. We learned that I had about one-third the optimum amount of vitamin D in my system and I immediately began to take supplements.

Within eight weeks after the surgery, the next part of the conveyor belt would begin: the radiation treatment.

I was assigned to Dr. O, a visiting radiology specialist.

The conveyor belt will continue until my appointment on the very last day of treatment when Dr. P will explain the purpose, the possible side-effects and prescribe the daily dose of medicine that I will take for the next five years.

Dr. Q will interview me after my last appointment before I am signed out. Then I want to see Dr. R, who uses lasers to remove tattoos.

When I finally get back home to consult with Dr. A to go over all of these test results and tell her of my experiences, I discover that she is leaving!

Each time I need a mammogram, or renewal for my prescription, or have another question, there is a new doctor. Within the next three years, the conveyor belt supplies Dr. S, Dr. T and most recently, Dr. U.

~ ~ ~ ~
~ ~ ~ ~ ~ ~ ~ ~ ~ ~

In late February, 2015, when I was sufficiently recovered from the surgery, I had one decision to make. In British Columbia, there are radiation treatment facilities in Prince George, Kelowna, Vancouver and Victoria. Where should I go? How would I get there? Do I know anybody in any of these places? Was there lodging? Would I have to stay for the full series of treatments? Could I go home for weekends? What are the estimated expenses?

I made my decision and in early March. Kevin and I met with Dr. O, the radiologist. "May I record our conversation?" I asked, knowing that emotions would confuse my hearing and memory. The doctor explained the facts, but seemed utterly surprised at my response.

"Let me see if I understand. You want me to aim a deadly force at the part of my body that offered life to my four children?" My hands were clenched. My face bewildered. My eyes beginning to fill with tears.

"Oh. I never thought of it that way," he replied.

What does he think breasts are for if not for making milk for babies?

As I left the room, shaking, I realized that I needed a kind of help that would not be found on the conveyor belt of scientists. I had seen a poster for counselling. I ran down the hall, burst into the office and spoke urgently to the receptionist. "I need to see someone. Now!"

The next available counsellor was Ruth. She was not on the conveyor belt, moving me along in an efficient manner. She made eye contact. She listened. She was willing to share my inner struggles. She realized that I was 'Me,' a real person with a whole range of thoughts, feelings, beliefs and battles that needed to be addressed. Tears. OK. Shaking. OK. Anxiety. OK. Rapid barrage of tumbling words. OK. Silence. OK. I did not have to attempt composure. She was capable of riding out the storm.

~ ~ ~ ~
~ ~ ~ ~ ~ ~ ~ ~ ~ ~

During the month of March, Ruth and I scheduled weekly telephone appointments. The intention was for me to have access to her through weekly sessions in her office while I was at the cancer treatment facility.

"I've decided what to do!" My voice was bright when we spoke on the telephone, so unlike our first time together. "I am bringing five disguises. I will print counterfeit ID cards. I plan to schedule *daily* sessions with you! I think one hour of counselling for every 40 seconds of radiation is about the right ratio!"

It was marvellous to laugh together.

The next week, I began again. "I have decided what to do!" I could hear her smile while she waited for my announcement. "I will pretend I am auditioning to be in a science fiction movie!"

"Sounds interesting!" Her voice was so warm and welcoming.

"The part I have to play is simply to lie quietly on this table surrounded by technicians in white lab coats, muttering multi-syllable words to each other while scribbling on clipboards. The set has space-age machinery, which hums, and clicks, and moves, and buzzes. Since the camera angle for the movie was important, I will have to audition, be short listed, then be accepted for the role and eventually have a total of sixteen turns on the movie set. That way I can pretend each radiation appointment is nothing. I could be completely passive and just get through the event."

∿　∿ ∿ ∿
∿ ∿ ∿ ∿ ∿　∿ ∿ ∿ ∿ ∿

Today, my counselling appointment is at 9:00. This is the first time Kevin will meet met Ruth.

"I have discovered another significant layer of why I am so frightened. Kevin is familiar with this part of my life. I just realized that a childhood fear is multiplying my anxiety to be such a dramatic, exaggerated reaction." I am so glad Ruth does not take notes while I talk. She retains a lot, though, because she is always able to recall my stories and comments, and help me untangle my own knots, follow my own threads, and help me connect fragments to become a whole.

"When I was small, my relatives kept talking about me, saying, 'she's just like Aunt Madeline!' I would overhear them whenever I was clever, or because of how I look, or commenting on my gestures and mannerisms. When I was four years old, Aunt Madeline was hospitalized for six months.[6] Two of my cousins came to live with us. I kept asking my parents, 'Is she having a baby? Is she sick? Was she in an accident? Did she have an operation? Will she die?' Nobody gave me a clear answer. When I was a teenager, I learned that it was a serious mental health issue. Schizophrenia? Manic-depressive? There were experiments with medication. Run-ins with the police. Electric shock to her head. 'Am I really going to be like Aunt Madeline?' was a thought that constantly haunted me. The Seer-church I was raised in put a heavy emphasis on hereditary qualities passed on to generations. Is it inevitable? Would I have a nervous breakdown? Could I tell it was happening? Stop it? Would I have frightening behaviour? Mood altering prescriptions? Electric shock to my head? Will people in lab coats 'do things' to me. Will I understand? Be strapped down? Sedated? Held against my will? I was secretly terrified of electricity, machinery, drugs, 'treatments.' What are 'they' going to do to me if it is discovered that 'there is something wrong with me?' And how will 'they' know if the treatments and procedures and drugs will actually work?"

"So, you have been worried about this for a long time," Ruth understood, "being diagnosed, being treated, being powerless and confused."

"Yes! Really, I have been rehearsing this inner turmoil without telling anyone for over 50 years! That is a long time to wait and see if something bad will happen! I have been looking over my shoulder to see if it is sneaking up on me. Observing myself. Cautious. Tumbling unanswered questions. Never asking! Never daring! Wanting to know more. Scared to know more." I pause. "It's not fun."

"How do you feel now? Talking about it?" Ruth gently nudges me to explore a little more. To focus on the present. I feel secure with both Ruth and Kevin listening to me. He knows the story. She has the skill.

I take a long, deep breath and sigh. "Actually," I check inside my body, scan my mind, listen to my heart, search for sensations. "Actually, I feel lighter. Like the windows are washed. Like there is more light. Like I have set down a heavy load."

"I can certainly understand why this whole situation has been extra alarming for you!" Ruth empathizes. "You have been assigned a very similar thing to the scene in your worst nightmare!"

"Yes! Electricity is invisible power. Radiation is invisible power. Aunt Madeline would have been strapped to a table. I have to lay on a table. Nobody could predict with one hundred percent certainty how her body and brain would react to the treatment. And she had reoccurring episodes no matter what they tried. She was in and out of the hospital right up to her old age. Nobody can predict the success of the treatments I have been recommended." I reach for my husband's hand. "It is pretty scary to submit to an authority figure without understanding exactly what is happening."

"You have made a huge self-discovery!" Ruth gently indicates our time will soon be up. "It will be interesting to observe your own awareness now that you know this about yourself. Old fears do not have to cloud present situations. The incomplete and possibly inaccurate information you had as a child does not have to govern your decision-making now as an adult. You are in a much better position to monitor your own emotions as they expand and fade now that you recognize the source."

I can see that. It is like I have climbed to a plateau and I can look down at my own life.

"Let's try an exercise," Ruth suggests. "Kevin, you, too, if you like." Kevin nods. "Suppose when the fear pops up uninvited, you speak to it and say, 'I recognize you. You have been here before. I have heard what you have to say. I don't want you to stay here now.' And then imagine the fear walking out and you can close the door. It will be so fresh and quiet and peaceful without that nagging pest!"

We practice a couple of times.

"I think that will be a big relief!" I know from previous counsellors that just talking this over will give me more clarity to 'close the door' on the unwelcome wave of fear.

～　～ ～ ～
～ ～ ～ ～ ～　～ ～ ～ ～ ～

At 10:15, for the third time, Kevin stands near while I lie on the table.

For the third time, I am alone in the room, holding the eagle necklace and ten purple beads, counting the seconds.

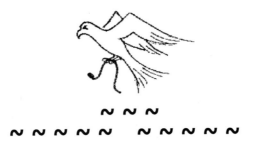

～ ～ ～
～ ～ ～ ～ ～　～ ～ ～ ～ ～

For the third time, I visit the marsh, send my Falcon, capture the eels.

For the third time I dress and exit.

But, this time, I am going home.

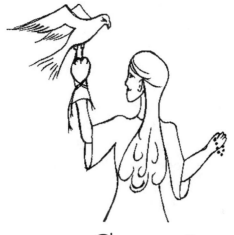

Chapter 3
Thursday, Friday, Saturday, Sunday
April 2, 3, 4, 5, 2015
Four Holy Days are all One Piece

What one man can do is dream.

What one man can do is love.

What one man can do it change the world

and make it new again.

Here you see what one man can do.

     —What One Man Can Do, John Denver[7]

~ ~ ~

~ ~ ~ ~ ~   ~ ~ ~ ~ ~

I feel like I want to build a fortress of teddy bears all around me. Bunnies and lambs and duckies and puppies and kitties and piles and rows and stacks of teddy bears.

I want to absorb the loving kindness sent by each person who gave me a token of our friendship. I crave physical reassurances to know that I am not alone. That I have value. That there are people who want to see me again. That I have an identity other than the 'Lifetime Cancer Identification Number.'

I am going home for a four day weekend. I feel like I am in a dream. Did it really happen? Does the cancer centre actually exist? Was it just a nightmare? Am I awake now? Is it over? Or is my happy home the dream? And a potentially life-threatening illness is the reality stalking me?

I want to burrow into some cozy nest and just sleep. I want to find a way to stop my head from whirling and worrying, wondering and waiting. I want escape. Not just from the physical situation, but from the state of mind I seem to be enslaved by. Cruel taskmaster. Sleepless nights. Exhausting days.

~ ~ ~
~ ~ ~ ~ ~   ~ ~ ~ ~ ~

Thursday

"It's Passover," I said, looking my counsellor straight in the eye on Thursday at our 9:00am appointment.

"It's Passover," I thought as I lay on the table and counted the radiation seconds at my 10:15 appointment.

"It's Passover," I said to my husband as we left the city, headed for home, zipped along the highway and crossed over the mountain heights. "I don't want to skip Passover."

But, it's a five hour drive, more with stops for groceries and errands. We'll be getting home late, tired. Kevin will need to light a fire to heat our empty, chilly home. Our children have grown and gone. How can I possibly prepare our Passover, Good Friday, quiet Saturday and Easter Sunday traditions under these circumstances? Maybe it's not worth it to even try?

~ ~ ~
~ ~ ~ ~ ~   ~ ~ ~ ~ ~

It's amazing how much information is layered onto one word. Passover is a day our family has been celebrating in a very particular way.

I love knowing that Passover is at a specific time. Not like other holidays that are kind of plunked onto the calendar without knowing the actual date. Passover is the first Sabbath, after the first full moon, after the Spring Equinox. Fitting the solar calendar with the lunar calendar is what makes the date vary so much each year.

We live at a northern latitude and in a deep valley where winter's darkness leaves barely five hours of sunshine on midwinter's day. It is significant to notice when the spring equinox restores the twelve hour day - night balance. Welcoming back the robins, Canada geese and other migratory birds, the sunlight signals awakening for every seed and bulb and twig. By midsummer, first daylight begins before 3:00am and lasts until well after 10:00pm. Completing the cycle, the autumnal equinox arrives with the twelve hour day - night balance. Then the winter solstice plunges us back into winter's dark. It seems such a long wait until spring's light returns.

Since we live far from streetlights, the moon's cycle is also noticeable. On moonless nights, familiar constellations are easily recognizable and the wide banner of the Milky Way splashes across the sky. When the moon is full in summertime, the stars are blotted out and the bright moon extends the long twilight and early dawn. When the moon is full in the autumn, I hear the hoot of owls, eagerly hunting after the leaves have fallen and before snow covers the pathways of their prey. When the moon is full in the wintertime, the snow reflects brilliant sparkles of white wonder. When the moon is full in the springtime, I can see across the river where coyotes howl.

Since we chose the 'Back-to-Nature' lifestyle, these seasonal shifts are significant. Not because seasonal holidays are announced on TV ads, or made obvious by the unavoidable bombardment of Mall merchandise, or demanded by social pressure to participate. The seasons are an actual reality. As a trio they dance: sun – moon – earth. And we go along for the ride.

Passover is a real time. It happened once in history, but is marked annually to remember something that needs to be retold, needs to be re-enacted.

An armed government rumoured prejudice, built up suspicion and enslaved a People, outlawed their religious beliefs, forced labour, limited where they could live, assigned occupations, prevented emigration. Those who attended the passage of birth, killed the offspring before the first breath. Doomed, the People believed a Saviour would be born to lead them away from this place to 'The Promised Land,' to safety, to freedom, to a place where families, and traditions, and worship would flourish.

The book of Exodus preserves the story. Moses is the long hoped for leader. Passover is the night to remember. During the last night of the last of ten plagues, the Angel of Death passes-over the homes of the People who have claimed protection through the sacrifice and blood of a lamb.

To the best of my ability, while our children were growing up, I have built family customs to mark this night. The People were instructed to mark their door frames with the blood of the lamb. So, we do, too. The People were told to be ready to travel, to wear their shoes and coats and eat in a hurry, standing up with their bags packed and belts tied securely. So, we do, too. The

38

People eat lamb and unleavened bread. So, we do, too. Making bricks and mortar was the unending task of the slaves. So, we eat bricks of cheese and mortar of mashed potatoes. Salty sweat and bitter tears were the sorrow of the slaves. So, we dip bitter green vegetables into salt water. The People were commanded to 'borrow' gold and jewelry from their taskmasters. So, we eat colourful mixed vegetables to symbolize the gems. The Promised Land was described as a 'land flowing with milk and honey' and abundantly fruitful. So, we eat chunky apple sauce made with raisins, sweetened with honey, served with a splash of milk.

"Why is this night different from other nights?" the youngest child asks. The Scriptures are read aloud. We talk about the plagues and shudder to think of 'the first-born son' who would have been killed during the last plague unless he was in a home protected by the blood of the lamb.

Carrying backpacks, the children follow Kevin to a place where we can walk on dry land in-between long puddles, like the People did when they passed through the Red Sea. We imagine the protection God provided, guiding them with the Pillar of Cloud by day and the Pillar of Fire by night. We shudder to think of Pharaoh's army smashed and drowned by the returning water. We celebrate Miriam leading the People in a song of gladness.

∿ ∿ ∿
∿ ∿ ∿ ∿ ∿   ∿ ∿ ∿ ∿ ∿

I have my eyes closed as Kevin drives us towards home. These precious memories both nourish my heart and make it ache. Our youngest children left home over ten years ago. Is our family tradition all in the past? In what way can I renew what is meaningful on this day?

"I can make a simple supper tonight. Even if we don't re-enact the whole thing, we can watch 'The Ten Commandments' movie and participate at least a little." Charlton Heston will have to substitute for our usual feast, re-enactment, Bible reading.

And, as we do, I realize in a new way that this is not just a children's story, not just a Sunday School picture to colour.

I have my own harsh taskmaster, my own sense of doom and monotonous plodding on a path I don't want to be on, a lack of freedom. I have been taken over by a plague! Where is my protection? My long hoped for leader? My safe haven? How do I get out of here? Is there a 'Promised Land' I can escape to?

I keep thinking that I am so weak, that I am 'wrong' and 'bad' to keep switching from courage to cowardice, from calm to fear. Why can't I just believe? Why can't I say 'Yes' once and then rest?

We repeat customs every year. Repetition is part of the Path. I am like the People who believe, then doubt. It is unrealistic to think that I will ever be without questions or entirely certain.

The People had just finished witnessing the Almighty at work masterminding their miraculous exit, and then, at the banks of the Red Sea, they doubt that God is even there.

This is precisely why this story must be told and retold, to comfort ourselves, that it is normal to waver, that God is the reliable One. The Psalms are filled with this reminder. I feel low, but God lifts me up. I feel alone, but God is near. I have turned away... again, but God is patient. I have done wrong, but God forgives. I am broken, but God restores. I have lost my sense of purpose, but God has a plan. I am afraid, but the Lord is my Shepherd.

~ ~ ~

~ ~ ~ ~ ~   ~ ~ ~ ~ ~

Although the full banquet is too much for me to accomplish this year, it only takes a moment to bring the flannel board figures downstairs and set up the scenes on the windowsill as we move through each part of the story over the weekend.

Thursday

Jesus sits at the table to share the Passover meal with His disciples during the Last Supper and instituted the new meaning of the bread and wine. "Take. Eat. This is my body. Take. Drink. This is my blood."

Friday

The Crucifixion. Once and for all, Jesus gives Passover a new meaning as He offers Himself as the sacrifice for salvation from the death of sin to those who ask to be protected by 'the Blood of the Lamb.'

I place the flannel board figures to create the scene. Jesus is wrapped in the tomb. The huge stone seals the entrance. The soldiers stand guard.

~ ~ ~
~ ~ ~ ~ ~   ~ ~ ~ ~ ~

"I'm going to get up to watch the eclipse tonight," I tell Kevin. And sure enough, between 3:30 and 5:00am, out of the western window, just before dawn, the moon slowly passes through the earth's shadow. The sun, the moon and the earth dance together. Powerful forces at work. I feel so tiny. Later, we enjoy amazing photographs on-line.

What a time we live in! Nature and Science. They can be partners. Nature and Religion. They can be partners. Religion and Science. Can they be partners?

Saturday

The tomb. It is a long day of waiting.

Sunday

Before daylight, I tip-toe down the stairs to change the flannel board scene. The guards have fainted. The angel descends. The stone is rolled away. The women approach. The tomb is empty! Jesus is arisen. Alleluia!

But, wait. What's this? A cheerful pot of miniature, wide-open daffodils has appeared! I didn't do that!

"Kevin?" nudge, nudge. "There has been an Easter miracle!" It seems unfriendly to wake him. But also unfriendly not to include him in my gladness. "The flannel board garden has come to life! Daffodils! My favourite!"

"I wonder how they got there?" he murmurs. In dawn's light I see his smile flicker before sleep returns.

"I don't know, but it is the best Easter moment I have ever had in my whole life!"

∿ ∿ ∿
∿ ∿ ∿ ∿ ∿   ∿ ∿ ∿ ∿ ∿

"Let's watch 'Ben Hur' today," I announce at breakfast time. I have no goodies to hide or find. Somehow stresses have interrupted the event planning part of my brain. Charlton Heston will have to substitute for going to church, fancy feast, family gathering, Easter egg hunt and a new springtime dress.

∿ ∿ ∿
∿ ∿ ∿ ∿ ∿   ∿ ∿ ∿ ∿ ∿

We have watched a lot of TV since my surgery in January. Yes, we still live in a compact, wood-heated log home, but we recently traded with a neighbour for a flat screen TV! The local government used to provide a satellite dish so everyone in Avola had three channels, but we recently installed our own dish and now we have the remote control to spell in anything we are interested in. Poof! We can down-load anything that is 'out there.'

January and February were filled up with 'The Beverly Hillbillies' and 'Bewitched' and 'The Waltons' and 'Get Smart' and 'The Andy Griffith Show' and of course 'Little House on the Prairie.' We also enjoyed favourite musicians, biographies and interviews, how-to programs and lots of historic, archaeological and travel documentaries. That was a pretty good escape!

Mike, the librarian on the visiting bookmobile, brought extra movies because he thought I might not be feeling so well. How very thoughtful! We have been well supplied with entertainment this winter!

Today, I use the clicker to spell in 'The Shroud of Turin' and we participate in Easter by following the history, theories and scientific data collected from what is either the actual linen cloth Jesus was wrapped in for burial or the most astonishing medieval fraud that no method of inquiry has been able to debunk.

"Science and Religion! Look at that! They can both inform the other!" It is a fascinating study.

~ ~ ~
~ ~ ~ ~ ~   ~ ~ ~ ~ ~

Meanwhile, I have an ambitious 'To-Do' list, and Monday is also a holiday. I have been away and I will be away, but I'm home now.

It's Spring! There's yard work to do! The flower bed needs to be dug up. The stone pathway needs to be weeded. The lawn needs to be raked. There's firewood to cut, haul, split and stack.

~ ~ ~
~ ~ ~ ~ ~   ~ ~ ~ ~ ~

Indoors, I have to unpack and repack. Laundry, food, a whole bag of vitamins and supplements. I want to take fabric to cut for sewing. I want to bring my prayer book and journal. I want to find a drawing tablet and coloured pencils. I don't want to forget my camera. Maybe having activities that interest me will help the time go by. I intended to bring the laptop so I could edit and proofread my first manuscript, '10 Days in December' but I don't think I will have the concentration. Besides, I don't want any cancer Kooties on my lily-white, young-idealistic, newly-wed memoir.[8]

~ ~ ~
~ ~ ~ ~ ~   ~ ~ ~ ~ ~

There's money to earn. I write for two newspapers. I just need to polish a local history article about old homesteads. Kevin and I have pairs of photos of old log cabins, comparing when they were lived in way back when, and how they look now when the cabins are falling in.[9] Also, I'm writing a column called '14 Economies for Tough Times' about bartering, volunteering, learning, do-it-yourself, family traditions and gifts.[10]

~ ~ ~
~ ~ ~ ~ ~   ~ ~ ~ ~ ~

I phone friends in my volunteer groups to catch up on the news. It is no fun to be away from the people and activities I enjoy.

Daisy comes over to make me a special tea. How kind. How comforting.

Kerry gives me a bracelet to wear to remind me that she cares, even across the distance. The flat, oval stones are not perfect. They're flawed. That's life!

There's mail! The ladies from church signed a card! Our son, Nicholas, and daughter-in-law, Johanna, sent a special necklace. There's a love note from my Mother. She and Papa will come to visit me at the lodge on April 13. How splendid!

An envelope from Fran[11] holds a card decorated with a bouquet of daisies, the flowers for our wedding!

Just a little note to say,
you are in my thoughts today...
...and every day!
Get well soon!
... and Hurry Home!
Love,
Fran

~ ~ ~
~ ~ ~ ~ ~   ~ ~ ~ ~ ~

While I am home, I want to do things I like to do.

I have decided to make three of the 'Talking Quilts' I like to design.[12] One as a thank-you for Dr. C, the surgeon, who was so clear when he explained everything to me. One is to donate to the BC Cancer Society in appreciation of the grant I have received for lodging. One is for the young Dad on the cancer bus so he can tell stories to his seven-year-old son. It takes about five hours to make one. Picture, denim, picture, denim. They measure a little over a meter square. Each one has a theme: 'Real and Pretend' or 'When I grow up' or 'Wild and Tame.' Animals, machinery, ecosystems, transportation, farm, mountains, I have collected over 300 different pictures printed on fabric. An adult and child can explore many topics to talk about. I won't get all three done this weekend, but I can make a start and, if I can come back home each weekend, I will have a project to continue.

∿ ∿ ∿

∿ ∿ ∿ ∿ ∿   ∿ ∿ ∿ ∿ ∿

I prepare a letter to accompany the surgeon's quilt.

> Dr. C,
> The first time I came to your office, without
> clear knowledge of my circumstances, and
> trying to overcome days and nights of fear,
> dreading the sound of the word... cancer...
>
> You were so thorough in your instruction, and diagrams,
> and explanations, and answers to my questions.
>
> Thank-you.
>
> The second time I saw you, the day of my surgery,
> I was quite overwhelmed by the myriad procedures,
> injections (thirteen needles in one day) and clinging
> to the security of my husband's presence...
>
> You were so kindly confident.
>
> Thank-you.
>
> In the operating room I was so afraid of the
> anesthesiologist (because my surgery date was so

near the date when my father died[13] from a serious
mistake that was made before his surgery)...

You explained everything clearly and I was not
at all afraid, trusting your skill and attention.

Thank-you.

After the surgery, I was so very thankful for your cheerful
greeting, which I conveyed to my friends and family:
"It is so rare that we ever see such a small, early cancer."

Thank-you.

In your office on February 5, checking the
healing, your feedback and observations and the
way you listened to me conveyed confidence,
which was so welcome after all of that fear.

Thank-you.

∿ ∿ ∿
∿ ∿ ∿ ∿ ∿ ∿ ∿ ∿ ∿ ∿

While I have fabric spread all across the floor, I also want to take
a look at resources I can use to make a banner illustrating my
Falcon hunting the eels to keep the marsh in a healthy balance.
Visualizing this scene keeps my mind calm every time the radiation beams diagonally across my chest.

I can stitch this eagle to the sky fabric I have. It is easy to find
mountains, trees and a picture of a winding creek in my fabric
stash. Before we left the city, I asked Kevin to wait for me while

I went into the big fabric store while I looked for something that could be the marsh... and I found fabric that was perfect for this project. I also have black boot laces to cut into sixteen small pieces to be the nasty eels. I will remove them one-by-one when each treatment is over.

~ ~ ~

~ ~ ~ ~ ~   ~ ~ ~ ~ ~

Speaking of 'if I can come back home on the weekends?' there are also a lot of logistical details to figure out. How will I travel there and back? Where will I sleep? Who do I contact for reservations? How early do I need to book transportation and lodging to be sure of availability? What food shall I prepare for my husband while he is home for a week? Shall I take any of my own food with me? Phone numbers. Calendars. Lists. Does Kevin have the information he needs to stay in contact with me, my doctors, my lodging, so he can be aware of any changes in plans?

"Kevin, there's no room on the bus! You'll have to drive me all the way there again!"

The phone rings. There has been a cancellation. I have a ride.

"Kevin! There's no room in the lodge! I have to make motel reservations! "

I'm on a waiting list. Suddenly there's room. I cancel my motel reservation.

"Kevin, Dr. O wants you to come to see his diagram on the computer, midweek. I have to phone his secretary to see if he can change that to the last day of the week so you can come and take me home."

Logistics!!!

~ ~ ~
~ ~ ~ ~ ~   ~ ~ ~ ~ ~

One of the hardest parts of all of this is what I have had to give up this year. From babysitting, to nanny, to volunteering in schools, to homeschooling, to Sunday School, I have been working for pay or as a volunteer with young children in educational settings my entire adult life. I have had to step away from the thing I like most of all. The pressure on our income for us to be driving to so many appointments, tests and treatments has completely overturned our budget. Ever since this whole thing started back in September, all of our gas budget has been used to travel to doctor's appointments. There has not been enough money to pay for gas for me to get to church weekly so I can teach the children. It's a doubly difficult situation. Not only am I deprived of teaching, which is the 'joy of my life,' but, because it is hard for people who live in town to understand, I get dirty looks when I do see them in the grocery store, as if I was a back-slider, or fake, and never took my commitment to church seriously. Just when I need encouragement, I face gloomy frowns.

~ ~ ~
~ ~ ~ ~ ~   ~ ~ ~ ~ ~

I have to double check our budget.

Somehow it seemed urgent to spend $300 on vitamins using the credit card!

I have to organize receipts to send in for a grant to help cover travel and lodging expenses.

~ ~ ~

~ ~ ~ ~ ~   ~ ~ ~ ~ ~

I phone family members who have shown an interest in my situation and offered encouraging support.

"Tell me what you think, Brother. 'They just want your money,' is a common conspiracy theory rumour. It's hard to contradict this mind-set." Yet another layer of worry I do battle with. In some countries, both standard and alternative treatments are for sale. Consumers shop for the products they think will work. My brother lives in the United Kingdom.

His voice is reassuring. "Because Canada and the UK provide medical services to their people, they want to spend money effectively for the best results. It would be foolish to use public funds for failed treatments and have repeat patients. Don't listen to the money talk. UK and Canada, in my opinion, have the best system."

~ ~ ~

~ ~ ~ ~ ~   ~ ~ ~ ~ ~

I have to type out a list of my supplements to give to Dr. M, the homeopath.

~ ~ ~

~ ~ ~ ~ ~   ~ ~ ~ ~ ~

I have to bake muffins.

∿ ∿ ∿
∿ ∿ ∿ ∿ ∿   ∿ ∿ ∿ ∿ ∿

And, I want to be sure to take time to print out the e-mails of encouragement. If I can't have a fortress built of teddy bears, I will construct a castle of compositions!

∿ ∿ ∿
∿ ∿ ∿ ∿ ∿   ∿ ∿ ∿ ∿ ∿

Highly valued is this e-mail from our son, Michael, who is in cancer research. He sent this message when I was first diagnosed.

Hi there,
Thanks for letting me know, Mom, and sending information. I do have a few things for you to think about.

Technical stuff
You have the most common form of breast cancer and in most cases early detection has a big impact on prognosis.

Trust the experts, but always ask questions, and only make decisions when you understand your condition, the issues and your options. Lots of people either think they *should* understand and are embarrassed to ask what they think might be dumb questions, or they think its too complicated to understand and put all their faith in the doctor's recommendations. Doctors have such a specific knowledge around their fields of expertise that it can be hard for them to communicate well with patients. Take it on yourself to be diligent.

Emotional/ Mental stuff
The commonly held belief or terminology about cancer is that you 'fight' it. (You hear people 'win' or 'lose' the battle with cancer.) I am strongly against this mindset. Throughout life the body develops in different ways and, just like grey hair, cancer is a part of the aging process for millions of people. Research and treatment have come a long way in the last decade and there is much work to be done. So, like I said above, understand the condition fully and make decisions based on solid understanding of options.

One thing I have to urge you *against* is getting caught up in the storm of alternative / holistic / naturalistic / remedies, diets, or regimes. I know you both have some wisdom and intelligence and are not the type to be sucked into scams. However, people diagnosed with a scary disease who are then promised a cure can make poor decisions in spite of themselves. The best thing you can do is maintain the basics of health. Healthy foods, exercise, rest and getting on with normal life.

Again, I appreciate you informing me. I'll be happy to talk through test results, medical decisions and help work through questions about the process.

Best, Michael

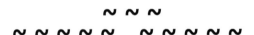

I keep reading the letter I sent out to family and friends in January:

Hello, Dear Family and Friends,
This is a message that is especially hard to write, but
necessary to share with my female family and friends.

First: clearly imagine in your mind the size of
a barley grain or half of an apple seed.

Or: go get a metric ruler and see how small 3mm is.
Pretty small...

So, now I will tell you why: In late September, I went for
a long overdue check-up at the doctor's office. One test
after another came back squeaky clean except one.

On January 2, I was told I had a 3mm size cluster of cancer
cells in my left breast. Later in January, it was removed.

It is hard to share this news because 'cancer' is an
especially nasty word on my mother's side of the
family... but... there it is... or rather... there it WAS!

Ladies, please take those mammograms regularly!
My overwhelming feeling is "I am SO thankful!"

My recovery is going fine. Kevin is a
wonderfully kind and attentive helper.

(gentle) hugs to all
Eleanor

~ ~ ~
~ ~ ~ ~ ~   ~ ~ ~ ~ ~

They phoned. They sent cards. They sent e-mails. I was astonished.
It is amazing how good it feels to hear kind words from friends:

Dear Eleanor,
Thanks for sharing your news even if it is not
happy news. Sending healing thoughts to you.
And yes, I have yearly mammograms!
Gentle hugs to you!
Andrea

Sending much love and sharing in your gratitude.
Love, Lori

Wow, Eleanor,
that is a scary thing to find, but so glad they did.
So, now... just healing? no follow up chemo?
I hate cancer.
It seems so unnecessary.
Love, love,
Lauren

Dear Eleanor,
I am so sorry to hear about your health issue
and surgery. I am glad you are recovering well
and have Kevin home to care for you. Wishes
for a speedy recovery and no recurrence.
Lots of love,
Liz

I hope everything goes smoothly!
Cheers, Dan

Be confident. You are more safe than the women who
do not go for regular check-ups. If you need anything,
speak up. You will be at the front of the line.
Bella

Kevin and Eleanor,
My wife had lumpectomy, no radiation, no
medication, so it came back and she passed away in
five years. So I say to you: throw everything at it!
Fred

~ ~ ~
~ ~ ~ ~ ~　~ ~ ~ ~ ~

In the same way that I took notes when speaking with my doctor
and counsellor, I decided to jot down and save encouraging
messages from cousins when we had telephone conversations.

Bella:
There is risk in anything.
I know people who hesitated.
Then it's much worse.
I don't know anyone who died from radiation,
but I know people who died
from not taking radiation.
Go to all of your appointments.
Just do it. Stop reading. Stop thinking.
Kill the cells!
Don't keep those cells one more moment.

My friend said, "I decided to confront this
or else it would be the end of me."
I am absolutely certain that you will be fine.

Kathryn:
Whenever I lay awake at night in fear,
I try to steady my thoughts.
'If I do this / don't do this, how will I feel?'
Maybe the Lord is using this to draw me closer,
to be more dependent on Him?
Take one step at a time.
I ask myself and my husband and the Lord,
'Help me to make a wise decision.'
I believe
that God has ordained doctors as healers.
They know the tests, and populations,
and percentages, and results.
It is OK to lean on what is provided.
Accept help.
I say to myself:
'I have chosen to put my trust in the people
who have skills and abilities beyond my own.'

Jeanne:
Recognize what's true. Reject what is false.
You did not somehow bring this on yourself.
It is not because God is not there.
There is not one 'right way.'
You are not 'bad' for struggling.
No one is judging
whether you do this well or perfectly.
Being human is being messy.
It is easy, but not helpful to think:

'If I could just understand (cause and effect)
then I would have done this instead.'
It feels awful!
There is no rest if you start thinking,
'What could I have done differently?'
It is not only one part of one body
– this is happening to all of us.
You can think,
'I am doing my part to heal all of us.'
You can see yourself as part of
this whole interconnected community.
You are on a Journey. You recognize it.
I love that about you.

∾ ∾ ∾
∾ ∾ ∾ ∾ ∾   ∾ ∾ ∾ ∾ ∾

Way back when I first started down this Path and learned what resources were available, I called the Canadian Cancer Society and asked for a Cancer Connection telephone buddy. When I described my situation, and requested a Christian buddy, I was paired with a woman who had a similar diagnosis and treatment plan and was a survivor of over fifteen years.

Louise is a trained volunteer. She set up a weekly schedule to telephone me. I soon learned that since we share the same values, so it was easy to talk to her. And I took notes so I could return again and again and benefit from her wisdom.

Louise:
Tools I use to cope:
'The Lord already knows.'
'Whatever happens, this is a do-able Journey.'
It can be quite a roller coaster of emotions.

One minute I am doing well,
then suddenly I feel overwhelmed.
First a spark of light, then unexpectedly,
something somebody says brings anxiety.
I decided to find ways to protect myself.
I believe
'I will be healed: through hands of science,
doctors and the Lord.
All healing comes from Him.
God is with me in the resources.
He will show me the path that
He wants me to go on,
therefore He will show me amazing things
along the way.'
People think you should 'take your mind off.'
But having cancer sometimes
takes over your thinking and time.
It's like doing mental gymnastics.
It is normal for your mind to go
around and around.
'Whatever I decide: I can never do the other'
(have or not have treatment).
It is normal to feel like
I can't trust my own body.
Sometimes, I feel panicky
if I have a back ache and lay on the couch...
is it coming again?
You will hear uneducated comments.
Don't allow yourself to latch onto false info.
Make decisions when you are level headed,
then follow through.
Then I think, 'If I worry all the time,
and then if nothing happens, what is the use

of wasting all of that time worrying?
We can easily think, 'I can never get through this.'
Yet, we cannot imagine God's Grace.
It is real. He gives it when I need it.
CLARITY WILL COME
For me, cancer was a warning.
The hourglass sand is running out.
Now, when I experience stress,
I stop and take stock.
I have come to have a softer heart and
I'm more open to hear so much more from God.
It is a Journey.
There are real lows that are tough.
But, there are also real highs
and Clarity, which is a Gift.

~ ~ ~
~ ~ ~ ~ ~   ~ ~ ~ ~ ~

Notes from telephone conversations with my counsellor, Ruth:
When I told her about the round-and-round-and-round
thinking all night she said: "Put all of these thoughts into a file
folder, into a cabinet or drawer. You can take a rest now and get
them out later. You can decide not to think about this."

I said: "I am experiencing unclear decision making, and difficulty sorting out my priorities: money (earn – spend – save
– give), time, church, fun, husband, house, hobbies, all of my
belongings, piles of paper on the coffee table and bedside
table. There is Christmas stuff still in a laundry basket so many
months later!"

She suggested: "Compartmentalize. It is not all one big blur.
Take one tiny action at a time. Do not negate what you are going

through. When a person experiences anxiety, they also have lower functioning capabilities."

I said: "'Meditation' is so often recommended, but I don't want to 'empty my mind' in the Eastern method. My telephone buddy is also a Christian. She said, 'Meditation for Believers does not mean 'empty.' It means 'with God' so I can listen, and rely on His guidance.' So that helps."

She said: "Here is one way to 'meditate.' Can you have a piece of clothing, object, person, phone call, religious word that is the key to stop the worry and return to calm? Recognize catastrophic thinking when it starts. Recognize your triggers. Is it helpful for me to go there? Build a story. Make a plan to have already in place so you have a connection to these good things so that when the thought/ fear/ emotion gets tangled and begins to get stronger, you can disrupt that, break away. You can deliberately make the act of interrupting it with your self-control. Say to yourself, 'I have heard from you before. You are not invited to stay here anymore.' Because, at this particular moment this is not helpful to me."

I told her the two songs I keep getting in my head:

Goodbye my friend, it's hard to die
when all the birds are singing in the sky...[14]

It's also hard to stop thinking of this one.

When ya comin' home, Dad?
I don't know when, but we'll be together then.[15]

Time passes. You can't hold on. A gloomy thought, but true. The only choice I really have is how I will spend this day.

~ ~ ~
~ ~ ~ ~ ~   ~ ~ ~ ~ ~

I write in my Journal.

My statement:
MY REALIZATION
MY BODY IS NOT ALL OF ME
MY STORY IS ME
THEREFORE:
MY DECISION, MY MOTIVATION, MY HISTORY, MY PATH
IS ME

MY ACCOMPLISHMENTS:
I am a married woman
a mother
a teacher
I have made over 100 quilts
I am a community volunteer
Brownie leader
song leader
Christian, catholic, music leader, reader
gardener
self-sufficient, back-to-the-land, 'homesteader'
homeschooler

MY CURRENT SITUATION:
A colony of cancer cells has temporarily taken up residence.
They have been removed.
I have been advised to follow up to kill them, because if there
is even one cancer cell left, it will re-populate.
I can only use the standard practice that is currently available
at this time.

I have decided to allow this.
I choose to also cleanse and nourish the liver, colon, kidneys,
lungs, blood, lymph, skin.
And to give a high priority to sleep, to provide my body with
what it needs to address normal age-related cell changes.
I continue to seek a wholesome philosophy, and
to live by my values, and to remain sensitive to the
Lord's guidance and protection and providence.

MY CONCLUSION:
God truly has a plan.
Eleanor is not in control.
He is in control.
I can cooperate.

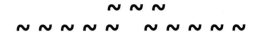

Treasure I found in my red Prayer Book:

> Give all who serve you
> the gifts of obedience and patient endurance.
> God is my Saviour.
> I trust in Him and shall not fear.

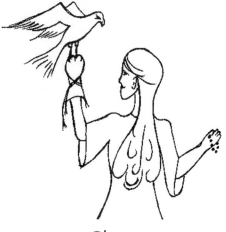

Chapter 4
Tuesday, April 7, 2015
First Day On My Own

Sunshine on my shoulders makes me happy.
Sunshine in my eyes can make me cry.
—*Sunshine on my Shoulders, performed by John Denver* [16]

~ ~ ~
~ ~ ~ ~ ~   ~ ~ ~ ~ ~

I cried all the way there.

As the bus carrying six passengers meandered between the hills, beside the creeks, threading past groves of budding birch trees, marshes thick with cat tails, dry grasslands, sharp rock cuts, spreading ranches, tourist campsites, the harmonious landscape contrasted sharply with the harsh inner-scape I had to travel, alone.

~ ~ ~
~ ~ ~ ~ ~   ~ ~ ~ ~ ~

To be at the bus on time, Kevin and I have to leave the house at 4:00am in the pitch dark.

The wood stove has gone out. My bags are in the truck. Every light is turned off. Feed, water, tie up the dog. Lock the house. Here goes.

Snowbanks line the driveway. As we pass the darkened houses of our neighbours, it seems like we live in a ghost town. There is no one awake to wish me well.

The headlights show snowbanks along the roadsides. The highway is clear. There is no traffic.

It is too dark to see the landmarks, but all so familiar. Smooth ice covers the marsh where generations of beavers built their lodge. I always look, because once I saw a cow moose with her twin calves marching through the snow. Above the wetlands, an eagle's nest is built in a towering cottonwood tree. Log cabins with leaning walls and broken-in roofs are silent now since the first homesteaders left after the paved highway was completed in 1969.

We arrived in Avola 1978 as newly-weds in our red and white VW van. For 37 years we have worked to make our dream a reality. But, this nightmare was not part of it!

I really mustn't speak at all. My voice will betray my emotions and I don't want to distract Kevin's focus while he drives.

It must be strange for him. He has been volunteering as a First Responder at highway accidents for 30 years. How many times have his interventions stabilized a victim? Soothed a child? Saved a life? His skills and quick action have changed history for families. Now, there is little he can do except get me to the bus on time and let me go. Others have the skills I need. Hopefully they can intercept the Grim Reaper.

"I don't want to go away from you," I quietly speak to Kevin, reaching my hand, asking for a squeeze.

After driving for an hour, beside the river, weaving through the rock cuts, passing dormant hay fields and pastures, near forest blocks harvested by logging, we come to the first streetlights. In this small town, at this early hour, no businesses are open.

Now long-haul truckers lead the way, carrying cargo between Edmonton and Vancouver. Kevin likes to talk to the truck drivers on his ham radio. Sometimes he gets weather information, or a warning about a lane closure or accident. Sometimes they compare travel experiences. Mostly they wish each other well with a cheerful voice.

Dawn comes. "Look! It's my favourite colour!" For a few minutes and miles, I allow myself the pleasure of absorbing the deep, rich blue.

"The radio is annoying. Can we switch to a CD?" I brought John Denver, a favourite since we were teenagers in the 1970s. I skip songs that are too energetic. I skip songs that make me cry. I stop the recording when I want to talk to Kevin or ask him a question.

It is 5:30am. Daylight begins. It used to become first light at 7:30 in the morning. We have gained a little more daylight every morning from December 21 until now.

Kevin and I are silent as we zip along the highway. It is two-and-a-half hour drive to get to the free bus, run by volunteers. Then another two-and-a-half hours to get to the cancer treatment centre. That's a long time for me to keep my emotions in check.

I try to push back the dread and enjoy the scenery, the mountains just hinting at green on the south facing slopes, the river winding, silvery ice outlining the shores, the sky clear.

"Look, Kevin! The moon is setting!" Dawn's early light is suddenly pierced by golden shafts of sunlight. "Look! Sun-rise and moon-set are happening at the same time!" I wish I could freeze-frame and hold onto this magical moment.

I am gathering in details of nature, of calm, of normal. I need a savings account to draw on later when I am away from all that is familiar, when I am alone.

The vision of the cancer treatments presses in on me. It is as though I am seeing double and not sure which is more real. The Forces of Nature? Or the Power of Machinery?

~ ~ ~
~ ~ ~ ~ ~   ~ ~ ~ ~ ~

Kevin likes to be early. Just in case. Train crossings, rock slides, car accidents, or highway construction are all reasons one might be delayed. We need to stop for gas. We could get a few red lights. Kevin likes to be prepared. I certainly don't want to miss the bus! There's no way to communicate with the driver. Very few people have those new cell phones.

We arrive at the bus rendezvous at precisely 7:00am.

We made it!

We wait.

The volunteer bus driver has just arrived.

When he unlocks the bus, starts the engine, gets the heat circulating, scrapes the frost from the windows, Kevin carries my bags to stow.

It's still early. Shall I wait in the truck, my heart pounding? Shall I hold on tight? It's so hard to say, 'good-bye'? Or shall I make the break, board the bus, claim my seat?

"You can go, Kevin," I have just about run out of being brave.

"No, I'll wait until the bus leaves."

Kisses to last a week.

I step away.

Now I wait over here. And he waits over there.

I cover up with an afghan, lean against the window, barely greet the others as they arrive, feign sleep. I don't want to talk to anyone.

I have already taken this bus twice, for appointments in the city, and returned the same day. Once to meet the homeopathic doctor. Once for the ink dots.

That was when I introduced myself to the other passengers. Everyone was friendly and shared their stories. Comforting? Alarming? I have never heard so many cancer details! What an education!

Everyone else lives near the bus stop, so they go back and forth daily. I am the only one from farther out-of-town, the only one staying all week in the lodge.

The bus begins to move. I wave to my husband. There's no turning back. I try to control it. But my breath betrays me. Wavering chin. One sob. I turn to the window so the others can't see my face. Slow, silent tears hover on my eye lashes, then, like raindrops on the window, find their way down my face.

I cry for the idealistic dream I am leaving behind. 'Back-to-Nature.' Growing our own vegetables, trading for fruit, butchering our own meat, all to avoid chemical contamination. Learning to preserve the harvest in the root cellar, freezer, drying and canning to avoid as much mechanical intervention as possible. Natural childbirth. Cutting our own firewood. Homeschooling. Working together on our property. It is so hard to weigh the options. Is there an 'all natural' choice for me now? Can I find it? I guess I am not a 'purist.' What ever other pathways there might be, I am taking this route.

I cry for the distance between me and every person and place that I know. I will not see one familiar face all week. Except Ruth. I sure look forward to my appointment with Ruth.

I cry for my fellow passengers:

Karen is a nurse who has helped so many others, now she needs help. Her cancer is similar to mine. She showed me her 'sunburn.' She is just finishing her treatments. She has been kind to me. She gave me her telephone number. Will I really keep in contact? Do I want to know how her future unfolds?

The slim blond lady beside me raises and trains horses. Her cancer is behind her eye! I don't even want to know how the radiation is delivered there!

A young man sits in the back seat. Derick has a seven year old son. He wants to use every natural remedy there is. He let me borrow a thick book with chapters by different practitioners. It makes me dizzy. Am I really going to search for and then swallow various sea weeds and other unusual plants? Give up sugar entirely? Cleanse my colon, liver, skin, kidneys, gall bladder? His cancer is someplace in his neck. His treatments are half way through. Last time I rode the bus, he was coughing blood on the way home.

Patricia, the woman beside him, was diagnosed at the same time as her husband. She forfeited her treatments to attend to him as he died. Now that she can start her treatments, it is probably too late.

Margie, in the front seat, keeps the music going. Sometimes the radio. Sometimes CDs that people request. This is her third time to be treated for breast cancer! An unsettling thought! The first time she had the lump removed, but refused chemo, radiation or medication. The second time, she had a mastectomy, and still refused the other treatments. Now she has it again on the same side, way down under her armpit. This time she is reluctantly submitting to the procedures she has avoided. Her story had a strong influence on my decision to just do it.

Once is enough!

I cry for my relatives:

Opa died from brain cancer when I was a baby and he was 54 years old.

Oma died from colon cancer at age 86. Three daughters and a son were at her side.

Aunt Anna died from a cancer in her lymph and bones and blood.

Uncle Otto and Uncle John were also taken down by cancer.

Aunt Ottilie most recently left our family. Cancer was discovered in the lung, but too near the heart to intervene.

Most puzzling, one of my cousin's children had a rare form of cancer in the pancreas. Seeking any new treatment, trying to hold on until his first child would be born, he managed to stay alive long enough to play peek-a-boo with his charming daughter, but left his wife and child so painfully soon.

I cry for all people who were undiagnosed until it was too late. All those who cannot afford treatments. All those who lived before science unlocked even a few clues. All those who suffered radical mastectomies before the spread of cancer was understood. All the turning points and decisions that might have been different and might have led to a happier outcome.

I cry, suddenly remembering that Father Sasges always wore the pink loop of ribbon, the symbol of supporting those with breast cancer. I never asked him who he lost. Oh, how I miss his kind eyes, warm smile, deep voice, gentle manner, careful listening, deeply reverent and sincere prayers, encouraging wisdom.

I cry for my friends who have watched a loved one hope, suffer, fade and leave.

Lauren was ten and her younger brother and sister were eight and three when their mother died.

Then, as a complete shock, her younger brother, Matthew, died at age 40 from stomach cancer, leaving his wife and children.

Sylvia's sister, Kathy, had throat cancer, leaving her with no voice, texting, even as she was dying, while they said, 'good-bye!'

Sandra's brother was only 23 when brain cancer struck.

Bill had surgery to remove his cancerous jaw and stayed inside for the rest of his life.

Jennie's life was cut short by cancer in her uterus.

Theresa had to make treatment decisions for her little daughter.

And Colleen's five-year-old sister, Khristy, died from cancer, casting a shadow over every five-year-old who came into the family later.

I cry for the families who have experienced death from breast cancer:

Kevin's Mom was eleven when her mother died.

Cheryl was only twelve when her mother died.

Allie was in her early teens when her mother died.

A lady at church told me that all of her five sisters have had breast cancer. She has had a lump removed from one side and mastectomy on the other side. One sister said, 'No' to treatment and died. One is an 87 year old nun. She had cancer 20 years ago. Here it is again. She doesn't want to have another round of chemo. But the other nuns begged her to stay with them. So she did.

Fran had a lump removed 20 years ago and did take the radiation. Here she is!

I cry for celebrities:

Walt Disney

John Wayne

Patrick Swayze

Michael Landon

Steve Jobs

Gone.

I cry for the chasm of loneliness. The lack of communication with my daughter and sisters.

I cry for the huge numbers of women I now belong to. The sisterhood who walk and run for cancer every year, celebrating their own survival, or the memory of those who have gone.

It is not because I feel sorry for myself. I cry because this 'one cell' gone rogue, has taken away so much from so many.

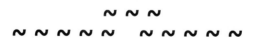

The bus arrives at 10:15.

I carry my luggage to the dormitory and check in.

A curved reception desk is staffed with volunteers who go over the sign-in and sign-out rules. The nurses' desk is visible through the glass wall. To the left is a large lounge with comfortable couches, a big TV and a table for puzzles. To the right, past the elevator, is a long hallway of offices and meeting rooms. There is a short hallway straight ahead. An all day - all night snack room with another TV is to the left and a small room with a computer and free long distance telephone is to the right. At the end of the hallway is the dining room. Two glass walls look out on the charming patio and flower garden.

Meals are served cafeteria style in the sunny dining room. There are as many as 36 patients each week. Healthy options are prepared by an energetic lady who obviously realizes that she has an important role to play in welcoming and encouraging each person in her care.

It is my first night in the dormitory lodging. I try to keep myself separate from this place.

I try to hear only enough to follow the basic instructions. "Here is your key. Keep it with you. Your room is reserved for one week. Your roommate has already checked in. There is the elevator. Go to the second floor, down the hall to your left, third door on the left. Your bed is near the window."

I try to see only enough to get to my own room. I don't want to see the wig room or the decorative scarves and hats for chemo patients. I don't want to see the daffodil lapel pins, the smiling volunteers wearing purple aprons, the inspirational slogans on the pretty posters, the artwork donated in the memory of patients who did or did not recover.

My key is on an orange elastic wrist band. The elevator buttons are clearly labeled. I see the right number and tap on the door while I turn the key. This is it. 'My' room for four nights.

The bathroom and two twin beds are to the left. A large closet and two dressers are to the right. A large window is straight ahead with a view of the lake. A bedside table beside and a soft light above each bed and a curtain in-between them offers some convenience and privacy.

My roommate, hairless and resting, offers her name and shares the information that this is her third time to come here for treatments. She will be here for the whole month without going home. She likes to read late at night and stays in the room most of each day.

I let her know that light and sound don't bother me. I get up to the bathroom in the night. I will leave the room early in the morning to walk to Mass. I intend to stay out as much as possible and not interrupt her reading or habits.

It only takes a few minutes to open my bag and load my clothes into the dresser drawers. I place personal things in the drawer of the bedside table: books, a writing tablet, tokens, photos and cards. I need physical objects to remind me that there are people who love me. I also have a small dark blue duffel bag filled with sewing supplies. Maybe I'll feel creative while I'm here with hours of unscheduled time. Maybe I'll write letters. Maybe I'll browse the stores. Maybe I'll walk along the lakeside parks. Maybe I'll find a library.

I have an insulated lunch bag with a freezer pack to keep my vitamins cool and I noticed a water cooler and ice machine near the elevator. There is a drawer in the bathroom for my vitamins and my personal things. There are two hooks inside the bathroom door, one for each of us to hang up our night clothes.

Everything is very, very clean. "Everyone here has a compromised immune system," I have been warned. "You cannot stay here overnight if you have any signs of a communicable illness."

The bed is comfortable. The bedspread, curtains and upholstery on the easy chair are an autumn floral. There is a telephone on my bedside table. Somehow that is very reassuring.

Near the elevator is a small lounge with a TV. I hope I can watch my weekly shows.

The other hallway must have more bedrooms.

Above the dining room is a library lounge with a cassette deck and CD player. Through sliding glass doors, a small patio overlooks the lake and lets in the sunshine and fresh breeze. I wish I could sleep out there. I wonder if anyone would notice?

~ ~ ~
~ ~ ~ ~ ~   ~ ~ ~ ~ ~

Last week, Kevin drove me where I needed to go. Now, I have to walk.

Last week, Kevin printed out the Google Map of the city streets. Now, I carry it with me so I can explore and not get confused.

Last week, we brought our own food to the motel refrigerator. Now, I have brought two bran muffins and an apple for each morning so that I can walk and eat on my way to Mass.

Last week, I had my husband to talk to. Now, I have to figure out everything by myself.

Last week, I had my husband standing just outside the door while the machinery cast beams of radiation through my innocent breast. Now, I discipline myself to get to appointments on time with my own will-power.

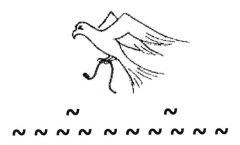

I lie on the table. My left arm is raised. My loyal Falcon swoops to capture another deadly eel.

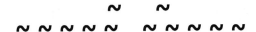

I do not enjoy the long, empty afternoon. I feel wooden as I stand in line for my supper. I wish the clock would hurry up. After I phone Kevin, it's bedtime.

Last week, I slept beside my husband, reaching out to touch him, listening to him breathe. Even if I lay awake, I was not alone. Now, I have to monitor my own night time hours. Awake or asleep.

Silencing today's bombardment, I lie still.

I don't want to replay the scenes of my day here. I want to replay the scene and enjoy the treasure I stored in my memory early this morning.

As Kevin and I approached the meeting place to catch the bus this morning, without the least effort on my part, a mini-miracle was given to me. Now I will draw on the savings account I made in my memory. Before I sleep, I will enjoy what I witnessed at dawn.

~ ~
~ ~ ~ ~ ~ ~ ~ ~ ~ ~

The full moon is sinking lower as we drive along. So bright on this clear night, there are shadows of the evergreen trees making stripes on the highway pavement.

Daylight whispers. The sky is glowing with yellow and pink. The forest thins and the ponderosa pine and grasslands show me that we are nearing an area of desert-like climate. The valley has changed. The mountain walls, on both sides of the ribbon-like highway which curves beside the rushing waters, have become hills that roundly rise and fall. The river is wide and slow. In this lower elevation, there is no ice. Spring comes here four weeks earlier than where we live.

Now Kevin has to concentrate. We approach the first traffic light at the northern edge of the city. Just as we pull to a stop at the first red light, three events happen simultaneously:

At that moment, the sun rises between the hills to the left, and shines its golden beams boldly onto Kevin's left shoulder.

Exactly then, a new song begins on the CD I have been listening to. It's John Denver's hymn to Nature.

Sunshine on my shoulders makes me happy.[17]

But, look! The full moon is also visible. It is setting behind the hills to the right. Enlarged by the atmosphere, its blue-gray texture seems to close.

And, I look again, intently, reading a message in this perfect moment.

Directly in front of us, a rounded hill is lit to the east by the glowing orange sunshine. The rounded hill is lit to the west by the silvery reflective moonbeams. I am seeing double. The rounded hill is much the same shape as my own innocent breast. The angle of the sunbeams and moon beams is precisely that of the mechanical mechanism, which beams radiation at my body. First from the right, then from the left. My eyes memorize this moment. Nature has provided an example for me. A map. A mini-miracle pointing the way, letting me know that I am provided for.

Time stands still.

How long does one red traffic light last?

Long enough for me to receive this gift.

Now, I hear in my heart, a verse from the Bible.

The sun shall not smite thee by day
nor the moon by night.
Psalm 121:6

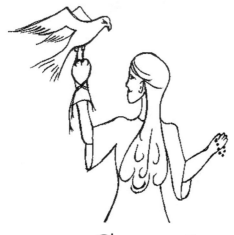

Chapter 5
Wednesday, April 8, 2015
Research. Resources.

And I'm looking for space and to find out who I am
and I'm looking to know and understand.
It's a sweet sweet dream.
Sometimes I'm almost there.
Sometimes I fly like an eagle
and sometimes I'm deep in despair.
—*Looking For Space,* John Denver[18]

~ ~
~ ~ ~ ~ ~   ~ ~ ~ ~ ~

My schedule today:
April 8, 2015

1) 8:00 Mass
2) 9:00 Homeopath
3) 11:20 Radiation
4) 1:30 Inspire Health
5) 3:00 Counselling
6) 5:00 On-line lecture
7) 8:00 Scheduled telephone call

Looks simple.
Lots of walking,
Nice weather.
But, I'm awake (as usual) at 5:00am.

My habit is to read the prayer book. 'The Breviary,' also called 'The Liturgy of the Hours,' contains readings for every day of the year. Priests have the obligation to pray eight times each day. This early Christian custom continues from Jewish practices to pray at certain times of day which are referred to in the Psalms. Father Sasges gave me this book after my Confirmation. I like to read it as soon as I wake up. It bridges the isolation and makes me feel connected. I quiets the rumbling anxiety and makes me feel safe and content.

But, today, on my first morning to wake up in the dormitory, snug in my bed, with just enough dawn coming in through the window, on an impulse, I do the 'open and point' method. Is God really there? Can He guide my hand and eyes to find a specific, helpful Bible verse?

I have my small, red New Testament with me wherever I go. I have been carrying it since high school. I used to wear it in the back pocket of my jeans. Now it is in my backpack in a small embroidered bag that my childhood friend, Liz, made for me.

The book is tattered. The bag is tattered. But, the continuity is soothing. There are lots of places underlined here and there, dates in the margin, an arrow, or happy face, or exclamation mark. Familiar. Comforting. Usually, I read in sequence. But today, it will be a random surprise.
Here goes! Open. Point.

For God did not give us a spirit of fear.
God gives us a spirit of power
and love and sound mind.
II Timothy 1:7

I'll take it! I want that! Yes, please!
'Sound mind!' Yes!
I want a sound mind!
And I know Who to ask for this Gift.
That was great. I want to do it again.
Open. Point.
Oh, Look! It's the Psalm describing the Passover!

God led forth his own people like sheep
and guided them in the wilderness.
He led them to safety, so that they feared not;
but the sea overwhelmed the enemy.
Psalm 78: 52–53

Led.
Guided.
Safety.
Feared not.
Overwhelmed the enemy.
These, I underline.

This is the God that the ancient Hebrew people and modern Christians believe in. The One who can enter time and space. The God who makes things happen. The God who made, and loves, and sees, and provides, and protects His people. And, look! The enemy is blotted out.

I am one of His people. Let me put my own name in there.

"God led Eleanor. She allowed herself to be led.
I am like the Little Lost Lamb. The Lord is my Shepherd.
He guided Eleanor while she was wandering,
alone, confused in the inhospitable wilderness.
God led Eleanor to safety.
Eleanor can trust Him and not be afraid.
The enemy cells that were inside her body are being destroyed.
The cancer will be overwhelmed."

I want to print this on a banner and carry it with me everywhere I go! And, I have so many places to go today.

~ ~
~ ~ ~ ~ ~ ~ ~ ~ ~ ~

My roommate stays up late reading and watching movies on-line on her tablet. She must have been wearing earphones, because I never heard a sound. The light coming through the curtain between our beds didn't bother me.

I told her I go to bed early and that I'd be up and out early. I planned my exit.

There is enough daylight for me to get organized. The door makes a loud 'click.'

I need to sign out and start walking before breakfast is served in the dining room.

~ ~
~ ~ ~ ~ ~   ~ ~ ~ ~ ~

It takes 22 minutes to walk from the lodge to the church.

My shoulder bag is packed with bran muffins and the apple that I brought from home, a water bottle, my prayer book, note-book, pen, ID card and dorm key. There's enough space to stow my sweater when the sun warms the day. Kevin printed out a map so I am oriented.

I call myself a 'city girl.' Because my Dad was a university professor, I have a lot of book learning, but very little practical, outdoors expertise. As a child, we lived in the mountains of Colorado, then in Florida on a short dead-end street backed up against the school yard. Next, when I was turning twelve, we moved to southern Ontario to a cluster of about 35 houses on half-acre lots surrounded by corn fields and forests. Since 1978, I have been living in Avola, which has become less of a town and more of a truck stop.

Red lights, crosswalks, morning traffic, cyclists, children, the elderly, poverty, affluence, the lake, the mountains, orchards, transport trucks, city bus, police cars, the mall, high-rise apart-ments and office buildings, gas stations, churches... it is a lot to take in as I walk this morning.

I call myself a 'city girl,' but I have never lived in a city before. While I am here, I intend to take advantage of every resource I can find.

Keeping an eye on my watch and the map, munching while walking, I feel small and like I want to cling to the earth. I whisper to myself, "It's my first day! Can I do it? By myself?"

Last week, Kevin drove me to Mass, so I am familiar with the location, building, sounds and sights. Before Mass, a small group gathers to say the morning prayers for the day. After Mass, a larger group stays to recite the Rosary. There is a tiny chapel with its own door where individuals come for Adoration 24-hours a day. One good thing about being Catholic, you can participate in these things wherever you go because they use the same order of service, call and response, prayers and Communion ritual. We are family.

This week, I deeply realize the value of this continuity. There is nourishment for my soul, no matter what I am struggling with. Silence. Sit. Stand. Sing. Listen. Recite. Pray. Partake.

I know where I am. There is rest along the Path.

However, I need more than the comfort of what is familiar. I am in entirely new territory and I need counsel. What do Catholics believe about science and religion? Some religions forbid specific things. In Ontario, the Mennonites did not use electricity, or engines, or any modern inventions. Other religions forbid the eating of meat. Some forbid the use of blood. Some forbid contraception. Some forbid war. Some forbid abortion. I can't figure this out by myself. I need peace-of-mind.

I go to the church office and ask, "Is there anyone who could spend a few minutes with me? I am in town for three more weeks to attend cancer treatments, but I am confused and afraid."

"Jean is here today. She is a hospice volunteer."

Jean is a steady, but kind lady with white hair. She looks very composed wearing a white shirt and a royal blue skirt and jacket. She invites me to a quiet room and signals for me to be seated. We are face-to-face.

"I am very upset," I begin. "I feel like I am telling God what to do: blocking Him from His Plan for my life. Is interfering by using science to change the process of this disease 'right'? Or is it 'wrong' to say, 'Sorry, God, I'm in charge of this. I am relying on the doctors, not You.' What should I be thinking?"

"What is the 5th Commandment?" she asks, then answers, "You shall not kill."

"Exactly! The surgery, radiation and medicine are all designed to kill! I have never killed any cells in my body before!" I am starting down that dizzy, bombardment of confusing contradictory ideas again.

"Sometimes a hospice patient confides in me that they do not want to take their medication, or they want to stop eating, or they don't want to finish a round of treatments," Jean's eyes are focused on me. She intensely wants me to hear what her experience has taught her. "If you reverse the commandment, 'You shall not kill,' you can see this, 'You shall do what you can to live!' You have a soul inside your body. Both are a gift. You take care of your body. It is a gift from God. Whatever is available, you use that to return to health and continue to live. We don't know what God has planned. We can participate in His Plan by appreciating and maintaining His Gifts."

What she says sounds familiar. I took notes while I was watching the Mass on TV while I was home over the weekend. "We are a resurrection people," was the theme the priest was explaining. I made a list while he spoke. Life is greater than death. Health is greater than disease. Love is greater than misery, grief, anger or fear. The Lord can cleanse away grief and sadness, anger and fear. He can cleanse away the harm and restore the good.

It made me think of how the Lord makes things live. He has made our bodies so that they can heal by washing away what has caused the illness. After the cancer cells have been killed, then I can trust that my body will rinse, cleanse, carry away the dead cells.

I am not trusting only in the doctor being able to kill the dangerous cells. I am mostly trusting in the Lord to be able to do something no doctor can do: restore a healthy balance.

~　　~
~ ~ ~ ~ ~　~ ~ ~ ~ ~

It takes 27 minutes to walk to the appointment with the homeo-pathic Dr. M.

Previously, I gave permission for all of my files and test results to be sent to him. Previously, we have communicated by e-mail to set up appointments. Previously, he has set my mind at ease with this message.

"Our best outcomes are a blend of natural and standard care. Think of it as if you are actually using two tool boxes. We used to say 'alternative' treatments. Now we say 'complementary' care."

He encouraged me to go ahead with conventional care, and that he could suggest supplements, which would make the cleansing and restoring part of healing go more quickly.

"Here is the list of supplements I am taking." A multi-vitamin, fish oil, acidophilus, fibre, and an old fashioned remedy. I also have three herbal options to help me sleep. "I tried to combine information from various sources. I also bought $300 of food-sourced vitamin supplements. Somehow, you just want to try to do something to help yourself!"

"This is a good start, I will add a few things that will also benefit you now, while you are having treatments, and other supplements for afterwards." I can see from the notebook of newspaper columns he has written, posters and brochures in his waiting room, and his clear decision making that he has had a lot of experience with cancer patients.

He gave me handouts about acid - alkaline foods and why to choose and avoid certain things. I am already using aloe vera gel twice daily on the 'sunburn' and calendula on weekends.

"I have a book about natural medicine and breast cancer," I want him to know that I have been doing a lot of research these last few months. I need to get as much information from him as I can during this appointment. "There are chapters on several topics that may have an impact on the probability of having breast cancer: hormones, the environment, toxins that come into our bodies from food and drink, what we breathe and touch, the packaging and containers we use, the lymph and immune system, nutrition, and also psychological and spiritual impacts, which might bring about changes in the body which leads to disease. I have made a kind of inventory of the possible hazards I may have encountered. Physically, I have made a point of healthy choices. I realize that chemicals have entered every area of our lives, so there is nothing I can do to become entirely 'pure.' But, I was wondering if you could give me clarity about this idea that there might be psychological or spiritual causes of disease, specifically breast cancer?"

I have two specific reasons to ask. One psychological. One spiritual.

Like lots of other women, I have my own set of psychological 'hang-ups' about my body. Bikini-clad, seductive women sell a lot of products on TV, billboards and magazines. I find this repulsive. I have had heated disagreements with family members about make-up, hem lines, hair dye and myriad other feminine products they use and I don't. Could it be that my alarm concerning this particular body part has set in motion an imbalance, which made an environment where cancer cells take hold? I know emotions impact heart-rate, lung capacity, and the digestive tract. Can emotions impact the mammary glands?

During the January telephone call with our son, Michael, I asked about this because he had been in cancer research. "There's not a one-to-one ratio, Mom. Think about it. You're not God. You can't make things happen with your mind."

And, as for the spiritual aspect, the religion I was raised in was based on the Scandinavian Seer's writings, which contained a world view quite different from traditional Christianity. This meant that for the first 52 years of my life, any Catholic or Protestant contacts I consulted would not be able to give me answers that would completely put my mind at ease.

The Seer reported a pleasant description of life after death in great detail. His world view included the belief that nothing happened on earth unless it happened in the spiritual world first. So, it seemed to me that even if I managed to dodge the illness physically, unless I addressed the spiritual cause, it would return. What could possibly be the spiritual cause of an ominous, deadly growth in my precious, life-supporting, milk-producing breast? Spiritual self-examination was becoming an obsession. Sifting through my life, looking for faults, and trying to decide what I should repent of, all of this anxiety was eating away at me. Worrying with no one to ask for advice made for a lonely, silent, heavy load.

Even though I did not believe the authority of these books anymore, I still did not have a world view to replace it with. And it was very hard to confide in anyone without sounding somewhat bizarre.

To make matters more complex, some of the local women I most looked up to had formed a prayer circle, inviting people with illness or chronic conditions to come for prayer. They had a book which enumerated diseases and matched the symptoms with spiritual causes! This physical organ represents this spiritual gift. So, this illness indicates a weakness, or sin, or flaw, or lack in this area of your life.

Invisible forces causing physical ailments? Strange? or True?

In John 5:8, Jesus said to the paralyzed man, "Your sins are forgiven you. Take up your bed and walk." Maybe that's where they got the idea of spiritual causes for natural disorders.

But, the opposite message seems to be conveyed in John 9:2-3. Jesus' disciples asked him, "Rabbi, who sinned, this man or his parents, that he was born blind?" Jesus answered, "It was not that this man sinned, or his parents, but that the works of God might be made manifest in him."

I have been wondering about this since early childhood. Why do I have freckles? Crooked teeth? Need glasses? What wrong have I done to deserve this flaw? What about people with serious disabilities? Chronic conditions? Life-threatening illness? I felt like I was walking in an eerie world, where unseen forces manifested themselves in distorted bodies.

I waited, trying to read the doctor's face.

Dr. M wisely replied, "You are asking questions that no one can know the answer to."

~ ~
~ ~ ~ ~ ~   ~ ~ ~ ~ ~

Walking. Walking.

I need to take advantage of many resources while I am in the city.

It will take nearly an hour of quick walking to return to the cancer centre for my daily treatment.

I notice a florist shop. There is time to stop and buy a cheerful bunch of orange and yellow tulips. Today is Karen's last day. She was kind to me while I was riding on the bus last month when I came for preliminary appointments. She and I have the same kind of cancer, the same surgeon and a similar routine of treatments. She set my mind somewhat at ease, letting me know that the radiation beam really made no pain, and opened her top button a little so I could see that the red 'sunburn' was actually not too bad. Since she was a nurse, she gave me a few tips about rest, nutrition and family matters. She gave me her phone number so I could chat if I wanted to share my experience. Those are very kind things to do, offering practical, reassuring advice to a newcomer.

∿ ∿
∿ ∿ ∿ ∿ ∿ ∿ ∿ ∿ ∿ ∿

I sign-in and go to the waiting room.

"Eleanor."

My name is called by a robot-like voice. Eyes down, silently, I enter, lay my shoulder bag and shirt on the chair, hold my purple beads and eagle pendant tightly. I follow instructions. I am left alone.

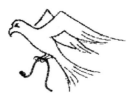

I count the seconds from click 'On' to click 'Off.' First from the right, then from the left. The door opens. I get up, zip up, exit. 11:40. Done for today. I lived!

∿
∿ ∿ ∿ ∿ ∿ ∿ ∿ ∿ ∿ ∿

I hear Karen's voice! I turn the corner and see her cheerful smile at the receptionist's desk.

The receptionist is the first person each in-coming patient interacts with. She is a tall, lean, efficient, woman who harvests information from her computer screen, but translates the data into a smile, eye contact and an authentically cheerful manner. She is also the last person to check with when each patient is finished treatment and ready to return to normal routines.

Karen is finished today! As I walk towards her, there is a flurry of movement. A few bystanders applaud. There is a little ceremony happening here. The receptionist is blowing bubbles, showering the departing patient with light-hearted congratulations. I give her the tulips. She likes them. Nobody knows the future. But, right this moment, there are smiles.

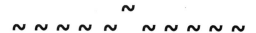

I grab a sandwich at the dining room to eat while I start walking again. This time, I have to go downtown. Beside old mansions converted into bed and breakfast suites, past apartment buildings, across four lanes of heavy traffic, cut diagonally through parking lots, into a small plaza, up the stairs, down a narrow hallway, into the office, ignoring the 'Do Not Disturb' sign, I enter a small meeting room.

The leader looks up, annoyed at my late intrusion. The participants have their eyes closed, relaxed, soothed by her voice. I take the nearest chair and without a word, imitate the others. I especially want to attend this lesson. 'Visualization' is a tool I am already using. I want to learn more about the value of this skill.

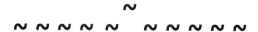

Last week, Kevin brought me to Inspire Health to sign up for the program which is a not-for-profit society promoting a new method of educating cancer patients in complementary forms of healthy options of self-care. I first heard about it when Dr. C, the surgeon, gave me a brochure during my first appointment. I also noticed the same brochure in the library at the cancer centre. The librarian told me that as of April 1st, the program no longer costs several hundred dollars to sign-up. It's free!

I learned that there are Inspire Health locations in the cities that have standard cancer centres, so patients can easily attend the services they offer. The information is also available on-line with recorded lectures and real-time participation in discussion or Q&A groups so I can stay connected when I am at home.

"I am not a bar code here," I had commented to the receptionist when I filled out the in-take forms last week. The holistic approach to health promoted by this organization is much more in line with my way of thinking. They don't discourage standard care, but encourage the many ways people can engage in various kinds of healthy choices and share information about up-to-date research findings.

I was given a questionnaire and workbook. I have access to four experts I can consult with. I sign permission forms for all of my records and lab reports to be accessible by Dr. N, the homeopathic doctor here. I feel hugely encouraged to discover that I can make appointments for a one-an-a-half-hour consultation with Dr. N and an additional half hour follow-up phone call, one hour with the nutritionist, one hour with the fitness person to design a personal exercise program, and one hour with the counsellor.

When I had completed my in-take forms, the receptionist gave me a schedule of weekly of classes I can attend. I was so pleased to see the list. Nutrition, yoga, meditation, art therapy, tapping, monitoring our own habits, journalling, and many other topics were available.

Last week I attended a session about meditation and relaxation. By following the leader's calm voice, concentrating on the breath and focusing on the sensation of the weight of each body part, I became very sleepy. I did not know that prolonged rest and deep sleep is a very important part of restoring health to the body after all of the cancer treatments. The body is working hard to take away the dead cells and build up the immune system. In fact, my on-going sleeplessness could be the most serious poor habit I have that I can somehow address and improve.

~

~ ~ ~ ~ ~   ~ ~ ~ ~ ~

Today's session introduces a helpful technique called 'Visualization.' Science has been able to measure the 'Fight-or-Flight' response of the body in an emergency situation. The chemicals released during this emergency response are not helpful to the healing process. 'Relaxation' and 'meditation' and 'visualization' now have scientific evidence backing them up as a worthwhile complementary healing activity. 'Prayer' would fall into the same category, I would think.

I realize that I have been frequently using this technique to calm myself and move away from anxiety.

Imagining myself in the scene bringing my Falcon to hunt the eels in the marsh is not just a silly fantasy. It is a powerful tool to lower the levels of cortisol and adrenaline in my body.

The scene of Moses with his arms held up during the battle has an additional strengthening effect because it is linking my mind to my spirit. My mind knows the text. My spirit trusts God. So, I relax.

I didn't have to imagine the special day when I saw the sun-rise and moon-set shining on both sides of the rounded hill. I can recall this pleasant experience at any time as an assurance that these beams of light are a life-giving part of Nature.

The leader has finished her instruction and passes out paper and coloured pencils to each participant.

It is somehow extremely soothing to draw the sun-rise and moon-set scene. While drawing, it seems I am learning additional symbolic details. A beautiful forest covers the slopes. It is a peaceful place. There is a cave of valuable treasure within the mountain. But liars and thieves have polluted the forest and contaminated the treasure. The sunbeams golden light banishes the dark invaders. The moon-beams silvery light beings cleansing. Order is restored and peace reigns again.

By drawing the scene, I have a physical reminder of the fleeting once-in-a-lifetime moment I witnessed.

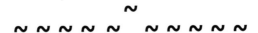

The world seems somehow softer as I walk back to the cancer centre for my weekly counselling appointment with Ruth.

Although I have been walking on sidewalks all day, I have also been walking past flower gardens. A corner church hosts a circular labyrinth with tall, soft grasses marking the spiral gravel path. An apartment building has landscaping of clipped hedges, flowering trees and white tulip borders to welcome the residents. A brick of house with a tiny elevated front yard brings hyacinths in full bloom close enough for me to enjoy their sweet scent. A street of older cottage-style homes has graceful willow trees just opening their tiny leaves and rock paths beside the meandering creek. More geometric, modern homes have zero-scape arrangements of rounded rock, potted plants or an asymmetrical ornament near the door. The mansion bed and breakfast welcomes guests with bobbing daffodils and bright red tulips in random clusters.

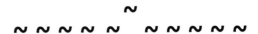

Ruth has opened the door to many resources. Besides her skill as a psychological counsellor, she has pointed out information booklets, introduced me to the librarian and suggested several organizations I could apply to for grants to help with travel and accommodation costs. She made sure I was aware of the resources I could access with phone numbers to the lodge, bus and the 24-hour nurse help-line. She helped me identify authentic on-line resources, too. The UK, USA, Canadian and BC Cancer agencies have reliable data and up-to-date information. Since I live too far away to participate in a support group, she suggested I make contact with the service that matches me with an encouraging telephone buddy. She runs a pain management clinic every week, sits on the ethics committee, and coaches families who are facing terminal cancer.

I am so glad that I felt comfortable with her immediately on that emotional day when I met the radiation doctor for the first time. Ruth and I have had scheduled, weekly telephone conversations during the month before the treatments began. She will be available to me for six months after this is over.

I am a fast talker. She is a fast listener.

"I'm still really bothered by the tattoo," I begin.

During the 'simulation' last month, when measurements were taken so the radiation would be aimed correctly on my specific location, I was told I had to have a tattoo to measure the boundary, so that the technicians could return to the same exact place to administer the radiation treatments.

"I was very upset. I absolutely refused the tattoo. I was shaking, and angry, and red faced, and crying, and my jaw was clenched, and I was speaking between my teeth. I tried to make it clear that I did *not* want to *ever* in my life have a tattoo, that it was disgusting to me, repulsive and loathsome." When I am anxious, I can remember the whole scene clearly.

"I said, 'A tattoo is for identification and ownership. It is for dogs and horses and prisoners. You do not own me. This is not my identity. I am not a prisoner here! A tattoo is for Auschwitz!' But she just sat there like a rock." It seemed to me that the room went dark. That I could hardly see.

"The technician would not consider any alternatives I suggested. 'Can we use a pen and I will not wash that area? Can I re-mark it daily? Can I come back for new marks just before the treatments begin? Is there any other way to mark the area?' I felt like I was begging!" My story spills out like a tumbling avalanche.

"She said, 'No.' I said, 'Then we have to call it something else.' She said, 'a permanent marker.' I said, 'It is NOT permanent. Somehow, someday I am having it removed!' I was so fierce!" I realize that I am shaking again now!

"It was really important to you and you felt like she didn't hear you," Ruth encouraged me to go on.

"Right!" It is amazing how wonderful it feels when someone believes you. "Plus, I knew that the other passengers for the bus to go back home would all have to wait for me since my appointment started late. There was so much pressure for me to be compliant. 'If I had wanted a tattoo, I would already have one.' I forced myself to do it. I felt like screaming when the needle delivered the ink. I am so against marking my body. No piercing. No burning. No cutting. No tattoos! I already have one mark: the sign of the Cross made with water at my baptism!" It is such a relief to have someone who will listen without trying to talk me out of my own beliefs, thoughts and feelings.

"It was a really shocking idea for you," she acknowledges my conflicting emotions.

"Imagine," I continue, "If someone said, 'You cannot have this life-saving treatment unless you do this immoral thing first.' What would you do? Do you see? Being forced to do anything that goes against my beliefs in order to receive life-saving treatment is a terrible dilemma, inner conflict, ethical struggle and moral agony. When I went home, I covered all of the mirrors. I hate those marks. EVERY DAY!!"

Ruth lets me rest quietly. I gather more upsetting ideas.

"It is bad enough to have the handling of my breast for the mammograms, strangers viewing, mostly men, measuring. It is bad enough to have the grotesque biopsy procedure, dye injected into my nipple, radioactive material circulating through my blood stream, and a total of 13 needles the day of the surgery. It is bad enough to be disfigured, scarred and wait to see if symptoms of lymphoma develop. It is bad enough to have tissue samples sent here and there, to wait for lab results. It is bad enough to read, and ask, and learn learn all kinds of new vocabulary, to study, and get conflicting advice and information. It is bad enough to have this long line of doctors assigned who I will never see again. It is bad enough to endure the pain and swollen, hard, enlarged breast after surgery. It is bad enough to experience the red, itchy, hot, breast after radiation. It is bad enough to wonder: 'What are they doing to me?' every single day." There's more.

"It is bad enough to be so far from home, without a friend, or husband, or family to share the experience with. It is bad enough to have to talk on the shared telephone in the lodge without privacy and under pressure while others wait to use the phone. It is bad enough to eat with people who are bandaged, red, hurting, weak. It is bad enough to overhear other people's experiences, worse situations, shocking realizations, more and more body parts, treatments, repeat cancers! It is bad enough to submit to repeated treatments, not knowing how things will turn out. It is bad enough to lose sleep, and worry, and be afraid, and try to understand, and have so many unanswered questions." Venting all of my confusion is a big relief.

"It is bad enough to have my budget destroyed, to not have enough money for gas to go to church, or see any of my friends for seven months because there is only enough money for gas to go to the doctor. It is bad enough to have the test before Christmas, wait for the results after Christmas and hear the word 'cancer' on January 2nd!" Will I ever forget the anniversaries of this experience?

"But, in addition to all of these necessary discomforts, and unquiet feelings, and unpleasant experiences, and imperative procedures... to have to give up personal beliefs and values, and cross the line to do something I do not believe in... It is such a tiny dot, but it is such an insult and injury to my character, my beliefs, my values. Surely, with so much emphasis these days on values and religious freedom, respect for diversity and preventing trauma to the patient, surely there is some other pin, or tag, or clip, or some other kind of ink that the body will absorb after the treatments are over. Surely there are others like myself who do not believe it is OK to mark the body." Now, I can make eye contact.

"You do have a point. If you would like to put this in writing, I can take it to the Ethics Committee." Ruth knows how to make contact with many resources. I am glad there is a way I can take action and a place where this can be brought forward as a legitimate objection. I feel a wave of gratitude for being validated. I don't feel like a crazy person. I might be different than the majority, but I still have a right to my values.

Unexpectedly, a smile flashes across my face.

"But then, this astonishing thing happened! The moment she pierced me with the needle, I heard this. 'A Pillar of Cloud by day[19] and Pillar of Fire by night.' God made a measurement. He set a boundary. He is a God of order. He gave instructions for the People to set up camp. 'Put this here. Put that there.' He gave precise measurements for the furnishing in the Tabernacle. The Children of Israel did not know the future, but they could remember and recount the things the Lord had done for them in the past. That built up their trust that He would continue to provide. The past holds evidence of God leading, guiding, protecting, planning! The Psalms recount from the time of Abraham how God promises, saves, provides, brings the People to safety. It seemed in that flash when she pierced me with the ink, that all of it applied to me."

~
~ ~ ~ ~ ~   ~ ~ ~ ~ ~

In the entryway, just outside of Ruth's office, there is a big display shelf of library materials for patients to borrow. I have time before supper, so I stop to look.

At first there seem to be three main categories of materials.

There are scientific books with photographs of different kinds of microscopic cancer cells, reports of research projects, and compilations of data with footnotes verifying the authenticity of each statement.

Less academic, for the purpose of educating the laymen, there are books and pamphlets published to give an overview in more general language so that cancer patients can understand the tests, results, options, side-effects and possible long range outcomes.

There are also memoirs and poetry, interviews and collections of first-hand experiences, and even humour.

Then I notice a fourth kind of resource. There are big drawers with rows and rows of relaxation / meditation CD recordings. Some are all music. Some have a narrator.

I definitely need all four kinds of materials. Curiosity becomes quiet when I read scientific facts. Clear, brief information pamphlets confirm what the doctors say. Conversational sharing connects me to others. Calming the 'Fight or Flight' anxiety may bring me a more restful sleep.

I need to evaluate my habits and set up a pattern of self-care actions. I need to collect resources, like building blocks, to continue learning and improving my health after my time here.

While I make a selection, I retrace the thought process I have taken so far. I have learned that cancer cells do not die. I have agreed to kill them using the methods that are available at this point in time. But, there is a lot of restructuring within my body that will be gradually cleaned up. This repair work happens best when I give my body what it needs: nutrition and water, fresh air and sunshine, exercise and rest. The science can destroy the invader. But I need to also trust that the Lord will do what only He can do: cleanse, heal, rebuild.

I sign out a sample of the CD recordings. There is a player in the library in the lodge. It only takes a few moments to tell if the voice and music appeal to me so that I can let go of tension. If they sound uncomfortable or annoying, then I feel like I still have my guard up.

When I hear familiar hymns, I immediately relax my shoulder muscles and jaw.

I will lift up my eyes to the hills,
where does my help come from?
My help is from the Lord
who made the heavens and the earth.
The sun shall not smite thee by day
nor the moon by night...
Psalm 122

I feel a sense of continuity to my childhood, to my beliefs, to the experience I had of the sun-rise and moon-set. Yes, this is what it feels like to relax. I do not acknowledge any physical sensations. I have gone to the sunlit - moonlit mountain to protect the treasure.

~

~ ~ ~ ~ ~   ~ ~ ~ ~ ~

Suppertime and the on-line lecture are scheduled at the same time. I have not had regular meals today. What shall I do?

The line-up at 5:00 will take a long time to move through. The dining room is open for two hours. I have time to do both.

The lecture is illustrated with diagrams of the body. I am reminded of something I learned in anatomy class in high school. The layman's term 'Fight or Flight' is more accurately named 'the autonomic nervous system.' The diagram shows how each organ and system in the body shifts when there is an emergency. When the emergency is over, it takes about twenty minutes for the body's chemistry to return to a healthy equilibrium. "We aren't chased by tigers," the speaker explains. "We have stress. At home, at work, social obligations, peer pressures. Even the media and entertainment can send a signal of alarm, releasing the chemicals in our body that shout, 'Emergency!' Often, the emergency is not over in twenty minutes, so the body stays in that state for hours, even impacting our sleep cycles."

Makes sense. Sounds like what happens to me.

"This sets up what we call, 'inflammation.' The body's immune system has to try hard to clean up the inflammation."

I have been hearing a lot about 'the immune system' lately. But I thought I was doing fine because I never get colds, or allergies, or tummy problems. I didn't know about 'inflammation.'

The lecture continues. "When stress or toxins or illness or injury cause inflammation in many body parts or over long periods of time, the immune system cannot keep up. A body in healthy balance can detect and remove a single cancer cell. But, now, cancer research is suggesting that an immune system that is overwhelmed cannot catch and remove that first dangerous cancer cell."

Now I understand why everyone is talking about rest, and relaxation techniques, and meditation, and soothing self-care. I thought it was all unnecessary pampering.

Too bad if someone else wants a turn on the computer. I need it for the whole hour.

~

~ ~ ~ ~ ~   ~ ~ ~ ~ ~

I also need to talk with my husband on the phone while I am in this noisy little room.

"Tomorrow is a big day! You're coming! We will meet with Dr. O, the radiation doctor, at 2:00 on Thursday. I've booked the motel again. My radiation appointment is first thing Friday morning. Then we can leave for the five hour drive home." I am so glad! I can only go home because I already made sure to reserve the bus and lodge so I can come back next week.

"What are we learning from the doctor this time?" Kevin asks.

"Dr. O will show us the computer simulation diagram. It's like a map of how the radiation passes through my body." I am a little curious and also a little scared to see the curve of my own ribs, my own lungs, my own heart, and the straight line of the radiation beam that passes through them diagonally across my oval chest and my round breast.

"I have prepared a 24 item list of questions to ask him." I hope to stay steady this time. "I'm so glad you're coming, Kevin. Be safe. See you tomorrow."

~

~ ~ ~ ~ ~   ~ ~ ~ ~ ~

The first time I saw Dr. O, it seemed to be hard for him to deal with my emotions. He didn't seem to realize that factual answers calm me down more than little soothing platitudes. When he said, "You'll be fine," that wasn't helpful at all, but actually made me feel stupid. Inside me there was a sudden flare-up of distrust.

I have to admit, it was hard for me to even hear his answers when I got emotional the first time we met. This is why I am bringing a list and taking notes. This is why it is so important for my husband to be with me. Kevin can retain the information and repeat ideas to me that are sensible. Later on, we can talk things over clearly.

I am terrified by the word, 'radiation.' I don't understand how it turns off and on and how it can be aimed at a specific place with a specific intensity. How can he tell if it is too much? Too little? I don't understand the impact this will have on my other body parts. Will they function again afterwards?

After the first time we met and before treatment started, I talked with Dr. O on the phone. When I tried to ask him questions about what radiation is, he was blunt. "You would have to go to university for more than eight years to understand the answer to those questions."

I understand the purpose is to kill any remaining cells that may have been undetected by the mammogram, that the biopsy needle may have seeded, that the surgery may have missed, that the lymph nodes may not have eliminated. I am haunted by the idea of 'one more cell' that could grow into a new cancer colony. How will we know if these procedures have been successful? What is the feedback loop? Who will follow up? Will I have more tests?

When I asked him, "How will we know whether the specific decisions you are making now will actually turn into positive long-range outcome for *me*?" his answer was not exactly comforting.

"If you're still alive in ten years, then we made the right decisions." His bedside manner certainly leaves something to be desired!

Only the holistic people are even talking about what can I do to assist in my own healing and possibly prevent any further cancer in all of these other body parts. The scientific people seem to be just checking off the boxes. They know when their task is done.

My mind zigs and zags like a network of rabbit trails. Every question branches off and multiplies into more questions. Partly because I am curious. Partly because I want to verify previous answers, cross-reference resources, and authenticate sources. I need definitions. I need to have some comprehension of up-to-date research. Surely there is a way to explain the basics in layman's terms?

A dazzling amount of money is funneled into cancer research. A dizzying amount conflicting opinions, hearsay and controversy abounds. A dismaying number of people are impacted by cancer.

However unsatisfactory it is to try to communicate with Dr. O, there are four other voices that have helped me steady my resolve.

Michael said, "Now you're into the numbers game, Mom. It's all percentages after this. No one can predict the future, only gather data from the past. And, although so much research has been done, the bottom line is: There is no for-sure-and-certain answer. What is the direct cause of cancer? How can it be completely prevented? How can it be completely stopped? Nothing is 100% clear."

His comments are straightforward, not soft, but somehow keep me steady.

Toby said, "Wow, Mom, just think of the medical treatments that were common in the past that are seen as foolish today. Maybe 40 years from now we'll say 'how barbaric' about this treatment."

This thought is very helpful. It feels like someone agrees with me.

Kathryn said, "Our pastor said that doctors are given a grace from God for healing. It is OK to trust your doctor."
Her faith feels like a sturdy banister I can hold on to.
Kevin said, "I do my best to help people. That's why I took the First Aid training. Doctors want to use what they have learned with great effort to help people. Plain and simple."
As always, Kevin's guidance clears my mind.

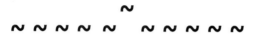

It has been a complex day. But, I am glad I stayed on my schedule.
There's not much left when I arrive in the dining room for supper.

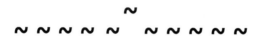

Back in my room, I surround myself with the comforting cards and the e-mails I printed out while I was home over the weekend. It is such a small gesture for each friend to make, and such a huge encouragement to receive. These people are resources I cannot run out of or be cut off from!

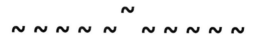

At the end of the day, like a cherry on-top, I have been looking forward to a scheduled telephone call this evening.
At 8:00 the telephone beside my bed rings. It is my cancer-telephone-buddy, Louise.
"I don't think I would be brave enough to do this without you!" I am so grateful.

I bring her up-to-date on the sequence of the week, the classes at Inspire Health, conversations I have had with my counsellor, Scriptures I have found helpful recently. I describe the mini-miracle of the sun-rise and moon-set.

"I made a list of wise words from special friends. I call the wise words my Stepping Stones... to get from stormy confusion to confident calm. I call these people my Choir! Louise, *you* are in my Choir!"

~

~ ~ ~ ~ ~   ~ ~ ~ ~ ~

Father Sasges
"Peace be with you" were the last words he said to me. Eleven days later, he died. This prompted me to get a check-up, which led to this early detection.

Tranquility
Between my diagnosis and my surgery date this word was my waking thought.

Psalm 105:5
"Remember the marvels the Lord has done." The Children of Israel never saved for 'tomorrow.' They only had enough manna for 'today.'

"Take care of yourself."
Mel said, "I didn't and now I'm in trouble...I just got back from chemo."

Eradicate
One word with great power. I carry this with me in my mind at all times.

Clarity... Grace

Louise said, "Clarity will come." She also said, "We can imagine scary things that might come. We cannot imagine the goodness and Gifts of God's Grace that will come."

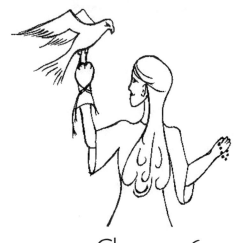

Chapter 6
Monday, Tuesday, Wednesday,
April 13, 14, 15, 2015
Visitors

I'll walk in the rain by your side.
I'll cling to the warmth of your hand.
I'll do anything to help you understand
And I'll love you more than anybody can.
—*For Baby, John Denver*[20]

~ ~ ~ ~   ~ ~ ~ ~ ~

There are some things you can only tell your Mother.

But I could not breathe a word to her when I first got the cancer diagnosis in early January.

In mid-December, my Mother had attended her sister's death-bed. Previously, she had already attended her father, then her mother, and now her sister, Ottilie. Each had died... from cancer.

I simply could not say that deadly word out loud to my Mother who had brought me life.

I found out about the breast cancer the same day that I bought a bus ticket to go to the funeral for Aunt Ottilie, just across the border in Washington. I stayed with Mother and Papa Joe. Aunts and uncles and cousins gathered. "Every death in our family is from cancer," Aunt Caroline, from Vermont, quietly reminded me. "At least no one has it now," Aunt Esther, from Colorado, tried to think of something positive to hope for.

But, I did.

My lips were pressed tightly together. I was there to comfort others, not draw attention to myself. My news could wait. Besides, I did not have any clarity about my condition, treatment plan, dates. I only had a piece of paper with words printed on it that I did not understand.

"When did Aunt Ottilie learn she had cancer?" I asked.

"April." And she died in December. I counted. Eight months. My tests were done in October, four months ago. It is a month before my surgery date. How rapidly is this unwanted guest multiplying within me? Without treatment would I have only three months to live? There is no one to ask.

I closed the door to Papa's study. I was on the phone a lot. I needed to talk to somebody!

Between guests and grieving and my withdrawn behaviour, there was tension between Papa and I. We didn't know each other well. It wasn't an appropriate time for me to share my burden.

∾ ∾ ∾ ∾   ∾ ∾ ∾ ∾ ∾

Besides the fact that Papa Joe had married my Mother, after she and my father divorced, and I knew she was safe, comfortable and well provided for, I only knew the basic facts of his biography.[21] I had been a dutiful daughter, coming to visit, talking with him briefly on the phone, sending greeting cards. He was retired military, a devout Christian, a man of generous and tidy habits. There was only one other bridge between us. I had given permission for Mother to read my manuscript aloud to her husband.

For her 80th birthday, I had printed off the manuscript for my first book, a memoir. '10 Days in December... where dreams meet reality'[22] describing the first ten days my husband and had I lived in the tiny log cabin we built in the summer of 1978 in the wilderness of British Columbia. Childhood turning points, our courtship, wedding, trip out west, and challenges we faced as a newly-wed couple included heart-to-heart details of my Faith Journey and how I struggled with the biggest decision of my life. Stay. Or. Go. When the temperature plummeted to -40°C and held there for three weeks, it made living in that cabin colder than living in a walk-in freezer.

My past interactions with Papa Joe had been pleasant and somewhat formal, however, I did not really know what his opinion was of me.

~ ~ ~ ~ ~ ~ ~ ~ ~

Dear Mother and Papa,   January 16, 2015

I have decided to write this and mail it so you can read it and respond after you get used to the idea...

This letter contains information for my female relatives.

It is the kind of news no one wants to say or hear.

And yet, it needs to be shared.

As you know, I went for a check-up in late September.

Dr. A, my new family doctor, sent me for every kind of test since I have not had a check-up for many years.

Each organ tested, blood work, Pap, x-rays, mammogram, ultrasounds and everything has come back with no illness... except one.

On January 2, I was told that there is a very small cluster of cancer cells taking residence in the left breast tissue.

That same day I left my husband to travel towards your home, to attend Aunt Ottilie's funeral. I decided not to say anything to anyone until I had more information from my appointment with the surgeon after I got home. You can now see why I needed to make so many phone calls and how private I seemed while I was at your house. It was strange to not say anything, but the week was not about me, it was about you and I did not want to add a speck to your grief and detract from your family experience.

I met with the surgeon for the first time yesterday.

He greeted me with the message that it is the smallest discovery he has seen for a year, that surgery (lump removed) and further testing of lymph nodes and surrounding tissue will likely result in no further difficulties.

Day-surgery is scheduled for the end of January.

It will be weeks to complete other tests and get more results.

I am in good spirits. I am glad I live in Canada
where our medical plan provides a high standard
of care and there are no financial obstacles to
excellent treatment and follow-up care.

When you would like more information,
we can talk on the telephone.

I expect no negative outcome, but a long, gradual series of
information gathering and explanations of the specifics.

The emotional swirls take more effort than
the actual procedures will take.

Kevin is strong and helpful. Our son, Michael, has
experience with cancer research. He and I have
talked on the phone so I can ask for definitions, and
compare information, and figure out a strategy.

It is a good time in the history of medicine and also the
time of my life to have a problem. There is an excellent
team available to me medically, and friends who care, too.

I am so thankful that I followed the prompting to get
that first appointment and found this so early.

Much love,
Eleanor

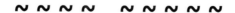

The mail was so slow! The letter didn't arrive before I had to leave
for the hospital. So, I had to tell Mother by phone! Not easy!

"Does this shake your faith?" she asked. "Some people say, 'Why did God let this happen to me?' What are you thinking? Feeling?"

"No, Mother. It's not that at all. The way I feel is harder to find words for." I am so glad I can talk to her about my Journey. "Here's the thing. When I was a teenager I thought to myself, 'I hope I don't die from cancer,' but if I do, I will just say to the doctor, 'Thanks for telling me,' and go home and let it happen." At that time, the methods of treatment were harsh and frightening. "I'm not afraid to die."

My parents had raised us in the Arbour Vale Church Community in Ontario and sent me for a year of high school to the Bonnie Hills Church boarding school in Pennsylvania. It was a different sort of church, following the 40-volume interpretation of the Bible written by a Scandinavian Seer. He claimed that he had, in full consciousness, repeatedly spent time in Heaven and Hell and had seen and heard people he had known on earth as well as historic figures. The Seer had described the experience of dying as peaceful and attended by angels. So, I was not the least bit afraid of life-after-death. Beautiful cities and meadows, greetings of friends and family, banquets and music, and worship in splendid temples; it all sounded marvellous.

Prolonging life didn't seem important, unless you still had young children, and mine are grown and gone. "It's hard to put into words, but I have this idea about death. Jesus walked towards His own death without making any attempt to prevent it. Maybe I want to be like that, too, trusting, not panicking." I paused to see if she could understand my thought process.

"So, why have you decided to go through with following the doctor's recommendations now?" Her voice on the telephone was hard to interpret. Without facial expressions, much of the message is harder to accurately receive.

"It's because of Father Sasges," I began.

~ ~ ~ ~   ~ ~ ~ ~ ~

Mother met Father Sasges, an 82 year old Catholic priest, when she recently came to visit me. She knows about how he has listened to my life story, offered me guidance and over a year of answering my many questions, welcomed me into the Catholic Church. I had five happy years of learning and participating, reading Scripture aloud and playing my guitar for Mass, teaching the children and attending retreats. Then he was assigned another parish far away.

As a happy surprise, he had just stopped in at my house in late July, 2014. We shared lunch. He gave me a handful of cherries and a blessing. "Be at Peace," he said and continued on his way.

Eleven days later, I had the phone call with the sad news. He had been airlifted to the Kelowna hospital after a sudden, extreme heart attack. He died in early August, on a special day when the Blessed Virgin Mary is honoured. All I could think of when he died was the simple prayer he spoke so often.

Jesus, meek and humble of heart,
make my heart like Yours.

I wondered how my life would be different without his kindness and wisdom to guide me.

The new priest let me know that he would be teaching the children, so I experienced a double loss. My Mentor was gone. My mission was gone. I felt pretty low. I had not needed antidepressants for the whole five years I had been going to church and watching the daily Mass on TV. I became fearful that the familiar, heavy, grey, inescapable depression might descend on me again. I decided to go for that first doctor's appointment, while I was cheerful, to introduce myself to the new lady doctor, Dr. A, so that she could compare my situation later if I became depressed.

~ ~ ~ ~ ~ ~ ~ ~ ~

I continued my explanation. "It's directly because of Father Sasges that I went in for a check-up. I had not needed antidepressants at all, not even during the winter for five years! Since I would no longer learn from his steady mind and wise heart anymore, I had been afraid I might slip back into depression. So, I went to the new doctor to introduce myself while it was sunny and I was doing fine. It's because of him that I have such an early diagnosis. It seems like a gift. When I see his picture, I remember that he always wore the pink loop of ribbon in support of breast cancer research. So, here I am." Mother seems satisfied with my explanation.

"You know, there was no cancer in the Garden of Eden," she shares her perspective.

"Speaking of the Bible," I interrupt, "that reminds me to tell you my other motivation." There are some things you can only tell your Mother. "While I was feeling low, before that first check-up appointment, I wondered what else the Lord might prompt me to do since I wouldn't be teaching the children at church that year. That's when I grabbed a pencil and paper and outlined each of my '10 Days' books. It was so sudden and so complete. It was like someone handed me a gift. I had a new purpose! I didn't think I could just say, 'Never mind. It's OK. I can die now!' It was an experience I could not ignore. So, you see, before I knew about the colony of cancer cells, the Lord already knew. He gave me both gifts: the prompting to go see the doctor, and the long range project of writing to give me motivation. So, although it is difficult emotionally, I have decided to go through with each part of the recommended treatment." My voice became quiet and soft. "It makes me feel safe in the middle of all of this confusion."

We were both silent for a moment.

"Your treatment centre is not to far from where we live. Papa Joe and I would like to come to visit you while you are having the radiation, if that is something you would like."

What a huge offer!

∿ ∿ ∿ ∿   ∿ ∿ ∿ ∿ ∿

Monday

"Mama! Papa!" I feel like shouting and running across the lobby and squeezing them both much too tightly. It is such a soothing balm to hear familiar voices. My eyes drink in their familiar faces, gestures, mannerisms. Yet, it is strange to have them here. Tender kindness and dear hearts clash with my own rigid routine and nervous anxiety.

They have come to see what I do here, and take me on outings. Hurrah!

We tour the lodge. Dining room, TV and lounge, wig room, nurse's offices, consultation room, and at the end of the hallway, the office where the volunteer bus drivers get organized. This is a hub city and buses come in from all four directions every day.

"We can go up these stairs so you can see my room," I lead the way.

I show them my treasures, greeting cards, books, sewing and drawing supplies. I show them the eagle and purple beads and explain their significance. I tell them about Moses holding his arms up to win the battle.

∿ ∿ ∿ ∿   ∿ ∿ ∿ ∿ ∿

I have to keep my eye on the clock. There are appointments this afternoon.

First: Mother steps into the radiation room while I get arranged on the table. For a moment, I am not alone! Somebody loves me!

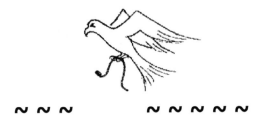

Second: I have requested an additional appointment with the radiologist, Dr. O. He was reluctant, saying that he doesn't have time for repeating information. But, I convinced him. "My Mom is well past 80. Every death in her family is from cancer. I am her firstborn. This is hard for her. She and her husband have made a long trip so they can participate in my care. You know my level of anxiety. It will be a great benefit to take this time so I can have their understanding and support." I stood up for myself! The world didn't fall apart because I asked for what I needed!

Better than simply meeting him and seeing the computer diagram map, Papa Joe asked questions to show his interest and listened for clarification. It took the pressure off of me. Since the emotions playing across my face were not confusing Dr. O, he was able to be present in a more straightforward, yet warmer manner and convey information by teaching and explaining facts much more clearly.

Tuesday

In the afternoon, Mother and Papa came to my third weekly appointment with Ruth, my counsellor.

I had previously explained to her that I have kept Mother up-to-date during our telephone conversations in January, February, and March. I don't know Papa well. There was some tension between us while I was visiting for my aunt's funeral. He didn't understand why I was always on the telephone. While I greatly appreciate his effort to bring Mother here, I am not sure how he feels about me now.

So, today, I am expecting basically a social call. "Nice to meet you." Polite chit-chat. "Thank-you for helping Eleanor."

But, there's more.

My heart warms and tears flow as Papa reaches for my hand.

"Eleanor, I want to ask your pardon for the way I behaved while you were in our home." He had previously had chilly interactions with me. Looking deep into my eyes, he earnestly continued. "I want you to know that as of today, I pledge to always listen if you need someone to talk to." His deep voice is so encouraging. "You must never hold back from confiding in me. I sincerely vow to be your Father in the role you need, both now and in the future, come what may."

~ ~ ~   ~ ~ ~ ~ ~

They took me to their first-class motel room. Papa went out to explore the area.

Mother and I had some 'Girl Time.'

Mother gave me a blue spiral bound journal. It is decorated with a silver bird, wings spread in flight. "It's a falcon," she smiled.

I show her my Journal and collection of letters, cards and e-mail.

I read this one aloud that I wrote to son, Toby, the day before the surgery. "I sound so confident and cheerful, but really, I was overwhelmed with emotions," I offer an introduction.

January, 2015
Dear Toby,
Today we are off to Clearwater for several
appointments, friends' hugs and cheer to
encourage me, prayer, massage, etc.
Tomorrow (Thursday) we go to Kamloops to sleep in
the motel so we can walk to the hospital Friday.
It is SUCH a small 3mm cluster of cells!
It is in a place close to the edge, no deep digging.
Minor surgery, for sure, and not a serious condition for sure.
It is such a small operation, yet I have waves
of fear, then calm thoughts return.
It is a great time to be alive for scientific help.
It is also a great time to realize the interaction of
emotions, beliefs, energy and nutrition etc.
It is a great country to be not one speck
worried about $$ for such excellent care.
Off we go.
Dad is steady, and gentle, and coming with me, and waiting.
We will walk together in the morning to the
hospital and take a taxi back to the motel later.
I like having a friend for a husband!
Dad is bringing the laptop so we will be able
to check e-mail as we move about.
Would love to open and see - read a message from you.
many hugs
and I love you so
Mom

~ ~ ~   ~ ~ ~ ~ ~

I show Mother my scars. There is a pale crescent line where the surgeon removed the cancer. He left tiny metal clips inside to mark the place that will show up in future mammograms. He carefully left very little change to the shape of the breast. The tiny scar where the lymph nodes were removed from the armpit is almost invisible. There is still a faint shadow of the green-blue dye from the day of the surgery.

"The area is still tender." I show her my reduced range of motion. "I don't want to stretch or lift yet. No jogging! Any time I bend or even walk down the stairs, I hold my breast still to reduce bouncing. How can I heal if there is always motion?"

She notices the red, clearly defined rectangular 'sunburn.' It is good to have a woman take a look. Share the burden. Even laugh!

~ ~ ~   ~ ~ ~ ~ ~

We drive to an over-look on the top of a mountain to enjoy the view of the shoreline and the farmlands and city down below. I can tell them a little of the history of the place. A Catholic priest came as a missionary to the Native People and brought fruit trees to the early settlers. The orchards, forest, ranches and outlying areas support such a big population along the shores of this spectacular lake.

They want to have lunch at the lodge dining room.

Mother walks with me to my appointment.

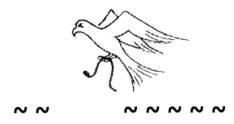

~ ~   ~ ~ ~ ~ ~

It is amazing to me that anyone, anywhere would want to stay near a person who is afraid, confused, suffering. I am so grateful.

~ ~   ~ ~ ~ ~ ~

Papa takes us out to dinner. We find a place that serves Ukrainian food that he remembers from his childhood. We enjoy perogies and sausage and cabbage served in a room decorated with traditional paintings and embroidery.

When we get back to the lodge, an old Esther Williams movie is playing. Mother loves her swimming and diving stunts, so we sit together for awhile, snuggled up on the comfy couches to enjoy the relaxed atmosphere.

"Lots of people retire here!" I suggest. "If you ever want to move to Canada..."

"Do you think you'll write about this experience?" Mother asks, "in one of your books?"

"My friends have already asked me that," I reply in a firm voice. "I told them, 'No way! I don't want to remember one speck of this time in my life!' They also said, 'Oh, you'll make friends and help people and have stories to tell.' I said, 'No way! I don't intend to listen, or talk to, or help anyone. I am going to walk in and walk out. That's it.' But, since I heard the word 'cancer' I can tell you one decision I have made about my writing."

I remember back to the bus trip when I went to the funeral, when I moved farther from my husband and closer to my Mother, when I carried the dreadful word 'cancer,' when I had no real understanding and a swirl of fears, when I spent a whole two weeks on that trip not saying a word about my situation.

"I was planning to use a pen-name. I knew that these memoirs would be built of my own personal thoughts, feelings, observations and beliefs. Talk about self-disclosure! But, I was also really concerned about privacy! I had a whole list of possible pseudonyms. Kevin wanted me to sign my own name. 'It's all true. It's our story,' he said." But, I was still uncertain.

"While I was on the bus, as usual, I struck up a conversation with a stranger seated beside me. As we shared places and interests we had in common, and while I was still wrestling with this new idea of 'cancer,' I decided, 'By Golly! I *am* going to put *my* name on *my* book. Who cares about privacy? I'll be dead soon anyways!' Which I don't think I will be. But, it helped me see the importance of leaving my story as my mark with my own name."

~ ~   ~ ~ ~ ~ ~

Wednesday
Mass

~ ~   ~ ~ ~ ~ ~

Radiation

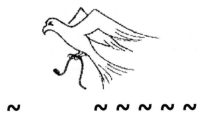

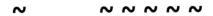

I am bracing myself. Now we have to say, "Good-Bye."

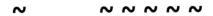

In my room, ready for bed, I look back over these special days. The comfort of my Mother. The dedication of Papa. The courage to step towards someone who is hurting. The wisdom to offer kind words. My husband, waiting at home. The future, always unknown. Each person has turning points and decisions. I do, too. I am on My Path.

Up, on a mountain, I can sometimes pause and look at my own life.

I hold this prayer card over my heart and try to find sleep.

God, I have no idea where I am going.
I do not see the road ahead of me.
I cannot know for certain where it will end.
Nor do I really know my Self,
and the fact
that I think I am following Your will
does not mean that I am actually doing so.
But I believe that the desire to please You
does in fact please You.
And I hope I have that desire
in all that I am doing.
I hope that I will never do anything
apart from that desire.
And I know that if I do this
You will lead me by the right road,
though I may know nothing about it.
Therefore, I will trust You always
though I may seem to be lost
and in the shadow of death.
I will not fear,
for You are ever with me,
and You will never leave me
to face my perils alone.
Prayer of Thomas Merton

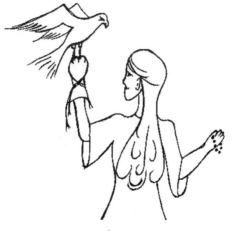

Chapter 7
Monday, April 20, 2015
Night Nurse

Talk of poems and prayers and promises
and things that we believe in.
  —*Poems, Prayers and Promises, John Denver*[23]

~ ~ ~

It's bedtime.

 Dreaded bedtime.

 I do so many things to try to get to sleep, but I seem to have forgotten how to do it.

~ ~ ~

The first week Kevin was with me. The second week was short because I stayed home until after Easter Monday. I was only in the lodge Tuesday and Wednesday, then Kevin came on Thursday and we stayed in the motel again and went home Friday.

The third week Mother and Papa came for part of three days.

Then my friend, Tammy came to take me for a walk on Thursday.

This week is my last week, but, I am here with no visitors.

~ ~ ~

The world is an empty place.

After supper (cafeteria style with salad, soup, vegetables, chicken, rice, desserts) in the dining hall (I try to sit in a different place each meal and not make any conversation) I phone Kevin (free long distance calls and internet in this tiny room right beside the dining hall with noisy people) and go upstairs (on the elevator to the second floor) to watch TV (in the lounge with three other people). I decided not to bring the hand sewing. (I do not want a quilt on my bed to remind me, "Oh, I made this while I was in the cancer ward!")

I fill up my water bottle for the night, scoop ice into a bag to keep my aloe vera gel cool. Third door on the left, I unlock my room. My roommate is in bed with her ever-present tablet. No matter what time of day I come or go, she is in the same place, reading or watching movies on her screen. Why is this her third time here? I don't want to know the details.

There is a curtain between our beds. 'Privacy.' Ha! I have kept a wall of silence around me neither speaking nor listening, to guard my own privacy.

I run a deep bath and stay until the water cools. The aloe vera gel is cool and soothing on the increasingly red 'sunburn.' I can now see the red rectangle all the way from my armpit to my sternum, from my collar bone to my lowest rib. Gasp! That's a large landscape! Not only the skin, but everything in a diagonal through my left side is damaged by radiation. Pause to look closely. I have been warned to watch the tender skin over the nipple. So far, so good. Look again. Inside the area of the straight-line sunburn, there is no hair growing in the lower half of my armpit. Wow. This is really happening.

I slip on my nightgown before I look in the mirror. At home I have covered all of the mirrors. It is too disturbing to look at my own body. I have to do what I have to do. Not wallow in misery again and again. It is not that the surgery changed the shape or size of the breast. It is not the scar. It is not the blueish-green dye injected the day of the surgery, which has still not entirely gone.

It is the 'tattoo.' I hate the tattoo. I loathe and despise and erupt with volcanic anger about that tattoo. One tiny pin-prick at the centre of the sternum. One tiny pin-prick under the arm half-way down the ribs. It is not good for me to see it when I am getting ready for bed. It will cost me hours of sleepless anger if I start to think about it. So, I don't look.

After combing my hair and brushing my teeth, I unfold the list and take my evening supplements and take three drops of an herbal remedy under my tongue. It is intended to quiet my rushing mind.

Oh, I hope I can sleep tonight. You would think the appetite for sleep would just take over, like hunger or thirst. But, no, it is harder than catching a butterfly. I get close and almost capture it, then, suddenly, an alarming thought chases it further away. I know the facts. 'Fight or Flight' is not the recipe for sleep. I have to monitor my thoughts and emotions. Tonight, I have a plan.

Cautiously, I stalk the elusive Sandman.

∾ ∾ ∾

The drawer in my bedside table is a treasure chest of beautiful, meaningful, reassuring items.

Last month, Sylvia gave me hand lotion scented with frankincense that she made herself. I allow her kindness and the indescribably soothing smell to help me enter a deep relaxation.

Opening to the bookmark, I slowly savour the evening readings in the prayer book that Father Sasges gave me five years ago. Knowing that I am reading this page on this day at this time with perhaps millions of others, I travel in my imagination to churches, shrines, homes, and people of all nations in prayer around the globe. I belong with these people. My muscles loosen their grip. I feel like a leaf floating down a gentle current.

Next, I tuck my little red New Testament and Psalms under my pillow where I can touch it in the middle of the night. 1974 was a long time ago. It has been my companion since then every time I travel. The Psalms tell me that every emotion, fear, doubt and dark despair echo across centuries in every heart, yet, trust in God's Providence restores bright security. I am not alone.

Also, under my pillow is the Rosary my husband found for me at Farmer's Market last summer. Hand-made with green agate beads, I have added a crucifix that belonged to Barb Liscumb and was given to me after she died nearly 20 years ago, and a locket with a tiny painting of the Holy Family. Mary held her Infant to her breast for comfort, nourishment and mother-love. Emmanuel: God with us. Christmas cards remind us of the sweet goodness He felt in her arms. Now, she is my Mother, too. I can take myself to this cradle and rest in bliss.

If I feel anxious in the night, I can reach under my pillow and touch these two significant Helpers.

Finished my bedtime routine, I stretch out on my back. In my hand, over my heart, I hold a heavy, small, red bag. I can hear the pebbles clink together as I shift my fingers.

Dianna took me for a walk along the pebbly beach near her island home nine years ago. The rainbow of pebbles I collected that day are in the red corduroy bag that Judy made for me when we were teenagers at summer camp over 40 years ago. A rough, red granite and mica chuck is in the bag from the place I grew up in Colorado. Clear glass, scoured smooth by the sand, is from the sandy shores near another childhood home in Florida. There is also a pink rose quartz, smooth, the size of a grape. Rose quartz is a symbol of friendship. When I hold this bag, or take out each pebble one-by-one, I can recall the voice and face, hug and acceptance I have experienced in each place and with each friend. Miles may separate, but the heart can connect.

Nasty! Invasive! While my imagination travelled, seeking friends, it also provided scenes of long line-ups at cancer treatment centres in so many places. Unwelcome thought! Ugh! Parades. Armies. Crowds of people. This ugly Cancer-Monster is destroying their insides!

Now I have to begin to calm myself again. Change the channel! Turn away. Slow down. A new attempt to return to calm. What else is in my collection?

Most precious to me are the ten purple beads I carry in my pocket and hold in my hand during each radiation treatment. Father Sasges made this little pocket Rosary and gave it to me two years ago when he was assigned to a different parish and moved away. It was hard to say good-bye to my 82 year old friend! I also have his portrait, a small card given out at his funeral only eight months ago. The thing that is so charming about the Rosary is that the purple beads on a white string were part of a long strand, like Mardi Gras beads, nothing fancy at all. Maybe he made a lot of these pocket Rosaries? He figured out how to attach the beads into a bracelet-sized circle by gluing a tiny wooden cross to join the ends of the string. The purple paint chips off of the glass beads. The wooden pieces he whittled are so tiny. The glue is somewhat lumpy. But, he made it. For me. I don't know what he'd say to me as I try to wrestle with all of my thoughts, feelings, beliefs, doubts, but I know he'd listen. I know he has seen many people through hard times. I know he believes that Lord can lead me, though I walk through the valley of the shadow of death.

It was because I was prompted to go for that first check-up that the cancer was discovered so early. So, when I hold these purple beads and think of Father Sasges, I gain reassurance that I am doing the right thing, even through my sleepless nights, swirling fears and stormy doubts.

I turn to lie on my right side. I brought a hard flat pillow from home. It is wedged under my left breast for support. It is a habit I have had since the surgery, three months ago. Shifting the breast still hurts. Holding still is better.

I reach to turn on the tiny battery tea-light on my night table, and carefully place it in the Christmas box from Aarti. Miniature wooden Nativity scenes have been cut, as fine as lace, on each of the four sides of the box, letting the golden light shine through. When she gave me this beautiful gift in January, when we met for dinner, I did not tell her that I was starting on this detour through breast cancer. She did not know that she was my fairy godmother that day, my Guardian Angel, giving me such a delicate object, which would convey so much tender love when I need it so desperately in the darkness of the night.

∿ ∿ ∿

With a jolt, my peaceful rest is jerked awake. The pillow under my aching breast has reminded me of another plaguing thought. I seriously considered a mastectomy. Even a double mastectomy.

'I could have done this!'
'I should have done that!'
This is not helpful inner dialogue at bedtime!

∿ ∿ ∿

Where in the world did I get the idea to consider a double mastectomy? That's a rather extreme response to the teensy-weensy dot of cancer that my original mammogram detected.

Angelina Jolie did it. During my first appointment with my surgeon back in January, he said a number of younger women are following her example. The thought process is pretty straightforward. 'If it's not there, it can't get sick!'

It is strange what happened next. Some call it 'Serendipity.' Some believe they have a 'Spirit Guide.' It made me wonder, 'Does the God of the Universe arrange so many details for my benefit?'

I booked a doctor's appointment in early March to seriously discuss this option.

While I waited for my appointment, I happened to flip to a magazine article. Somehow a researcher had measured a woman jogging. Her breast bounced up and down at 45 miles per hour! Yipes!

I started to list my friends who are flat-chested, who look great. Besides, many athletes are flat-chested and much to be admired: swimmers, ballerinas, models, gymnasts. If I did do it, I could just get bulky clothing, wear scarves, choose smocking, and ruffles, and shawl collars, or, decide that straight lines are OK.

While I was in the waiting room, one after another, I met friends who could help me think this through.

Two ladies I knew from the Quilting Club came in. "She has serious lymphoma. It is difficult to stop the swelling and pain," my friend explained, "since her breast surgery."

Right then Fran came into the waiting room. I have been following her homesteading advice since the day we arrived when I was 20 years old! I explained my situation and asked her, "You had a lumpectomy. How long ago was that? Did you have more problems? What made you agree to do the radiation?"

"Oh, well, I don't remember when it was. Maybe fifteen, no, maybe twenty years ago." Fran replied. "I've had no problems since." It was so comforting to hear her warm, familiar voice and make eye contact with someone who cares about me. "As you know, I don't really have 'a religion,' but I do have 'faith.' I just decided, 'They know more than I do' and I kept telling myself, 'It will all work out' and it did! I'm not one for worrying!" Those twinkling blue eyes! She's nearly 90! I collected my favourite hug!

My name was called. Dr. A gave advice. "If you have a mastectomy, the lymph nodes are also removed. This can lead to big problems for life." Her face told me that she didn't agree with my idea.

As I left the building, as if on cue, I met up with a couple that we are friends with through Kevin's Search and Rescue team. I knew they had had on-going health problems, so, when we got outside, I asked them about their experience with decision making. There's no one who can definitively tell you what is the best thing to do or not do.

"It takes time," Kevin's friend began. "We decided from the start to trust the doctor. No running around for conflicting advice and opinions."

"The hardest part for me," his wife said, "was deciding when to keep going? when to stop?"

As if I was in a play and entrances were perfectly timed, the next person I saw in the parking lot was the Brownie leader I had worked with when our children were small. I needed a ride, she had time, we had a conversation.

"You know me," I began. "I'm the Nature Girl! And I try to do what ever I do in a deliberate and ethical way. I keep thinking of all those uplifting things we sing and teach the girls in Girl Guides.[24] How can they help me make decisions now?"

We recalled several good memories. She encouraged me with her own health related stories. I recited the Brownie Promise I learned in Colorado 50 years ago:

> On my honour I will try
> to do my duty to God and my country,
> to help other people every day,
> especially those at home.
>
> *Brownie Promise, USA, 1965*

"I still live by that. No matter what storms or doubts come along, I can usually choose a path with this as my guide. How does it apply now? This is about 'Me,' not God, my country or other people... what is my duty to me?" It sounds kind of obvious when I say it that way. "Is it selfish to be the centre of all this attention? This expense? Is it 'my duty' to put my own needs first?"

"Well," she got straight to the point, "You can't do your duty to anyone if you're dead!"

That was helpful!

~ ~ ~

I phoned Dr. O, the radiation specialist. "I need time off. I can't think about this every day."

"You can wait four weeks to decide," he offered. "I will be gone by then. You will be assigned a different radiologist."

That made me dizzy again. My Dad's open-heart surgery was rescheduled. He was assigned different attendants. He died because of an error made before the surgery began. Would it have been a different outcome if he had kept the original date?

I am in a labyrinth with no way out.

~ ~ ~

It is 11:00. I have been tossing and turning for two hours. My roommate has just turned off her light. I decide to take a bathroom break before she is asleep.

Back in bed, history is the next topic my active mind provides.

~ ~ ~

Although I was advised not to go snooping around on-line for cancer web sites, one day, Kevin was away all day and I couldn't resist the temptation. From 3:00-10:00pm I clicked and read and scrolled and filled my head with pictures, graphs, interviews, statistics, recommendations, medical terminology and diagrams. I looked up the names of natural remedies. I compared the British, American and Canadian breast cancer pages. Some of it was review. Cross-referencing confirmed what I had learned elsewhere. I felt more a confident trust in my doctors.

Then I came to a history page.

It was fascinating.

In the 1970s several things happened that propelled the incentive to focus attention on breast cancer research. Women were holding public office. Women were in the military. Celebrity women weren't just pretty faces. Women stood up for equal rights and equal pay. When breast cancer struck Shirley Temple Black, she spoke up. In 1974, after her mastectomy, Betty Ford, the vice-president's wife, used her voice to raise awareness about breast cancer. A model posed in a luxurious gown on the cover of a major magazine, exposing the scars and the absence of her breast. Grants intended for medical research after the Vietnam War became available to study the condition of women. Because the spread of cancer was not understood, previously the standard was to address breast cancer with radical mastectomies.

Soon public figures and public fund raisers began the evolution towards the treatments we have today.

The research I did that day became stepping stones I could rely on to get me across the raging rapids when fears tackled my mind. Logic. That's the key. Put out the grass fires. Silence the clamouring.

~ ~ ~

Still. No sleep. It's past midnight. I have been here so many times. What else can I try to do to help myself? Shall I tip-toe out to the lounge and watch TV? Find a book in the library at the end of the hall? Go turn on the computer downstairs? Scroll through amusing pictures and stories?

Shall I call my husband?

Instantly: tears.

Oh, wow. I don't want to start to cry all alone in the night. Too hard. No escape.

~ ~ ~

But, wait. I have a good idea.

Pulling on my robe, I grab my Journal and a pen and make my way downstairs. The night nurse! A real person! She's awake! I don't have to be alone!

"Hi!" I fake a smile. "No emergency. But, I can't sleep. Every thought either makes me fill with fear or overflow with tears. Not a fun way to spend so many hours. It's part of your job to listen to people cry, right? Can I unpack my worries with you?"

She's about my age, a little shorter, a little rounder, dyed blond. Her friendly smile greets me.

"Have a seat. I was just making tea," she offers. There's a box of tissues handy. I might not be the first person to come to this office during the wee-hours.

The whole thing about making tea is that is slows you down. It's familiar. Safe. You've probably had a few happy experiences with a cup of tea warming your hands. I wrap up in an afghan. This lady doesn't have her hand on the door knob, pressuring me to leave.

After a few pleasantries and a summary of my situation, I realize why I brought my Journal. I can give her a tour of my head. Then, maybe she can help me find my way out of this jungle.

"You've seen these Journals?" Plain. Beige. Spiral bound. The volunteers pass them out to incoming patients. "I didn't want it. Who would want to remember this? Not me! I did not use it for many days. Then, I grabbed it while waiting for an appointment. I started to list things, not about cancer, but about the Lord. Things that happened that were perfectly timed. I didn't make them happen." I have no idea whether this lady cares a penny about God, but, I know it is not her job to comment or advise. I just want someone who will listen. "I think I'm past 180 items now. I don't write the sequence of the day. I just jot down what pops into my mind. Coincidences that I notice."

I open to the most recent entry. "I can't get the idea of 'Agent Orange' out of my mind. The jungle stripped bare. The children burned, running, blind. Is that what is happening inside my body?" I look up from my scribbles. "See? It's not fun to lie awake with thoughts like that!"

"I should say not!" She seems interested.

"Here are some pages I wrote about numbers, statistics and percentages." I read it all. Alone, these things loom large. Spoken, they shrink to more manageable proportions.

∿ ∿ ∿

a) I like feeling like I am an individual: now my data is tossed into the mix and becomes part of the statistics... blurred, nameless, without a story, path, no connection to a decision process or belief system.

b) statistics make me feel HUGELY pressured to copy everyone else (not a path I usually take).

c) graphs, median, mean, average, percentages is a combination of the singular... does not represent any one person, but rounds up or down to a nonexistent thing, then claims to be a reality.

d) I am not obese, a smoker, of an advanced age, already facing other health issues, so many, many factors I am not, so why would those stats have anything to do with my individual situation? 3.5mm is not 2cm or 5cm or any other thing... so stats for those things are not an accurate guide for me.

e1) I get the unspoken message: 'you'd be an idiot not to...' do such and such.

e2) and if I ask questions, the doctor who was assigned to me gets uncomfortable, makes it seem like I think he is an idiot... not good communication for sure.

f) at the cancer centre, I felt like I was walking into a funnel, the vortex sucking me into the no-exit hallways, the lemmings all leaping off in front of me, blindfolded, surging, hopeful of what ever 'the doctor said,' fear chasing along behind, the wolf of death snapping at everyone's heels, the faces in hallways, with little silent eyes down, polite smiles hiding terrified insides.

g) white lab coats with clipboards and numbers making changes to my body, which I dread and reject and loathe because the percentages made me do it.

h) no one measures the agony, no one cares about me as a person, no one wants to know my story, loss, views, hopes, pain, decision-making process.

j) just hop up on the table and allow numbers of grey, to aim at numbers of body measurements, for numbers of seconds, for numbers of fractions, until all of the boxes have check-marks in them and the stats can be added into the percentages!

h) questions, feelings, emotions are an interruption, a waste of numbers of seconds

>>>the doctor had his hand on the door knob!!!<<<

i) next I am expected to swallow stuff for a huge number of days, with a percentage of possible side effects from mild to life-threatening, which has a percentage of possible prevention of recurrence, no guarantees to actually work.

j) and all of this is to add to their stats, which will show I either lived, or re-occurred, or died in 5 years... or maybe lived, or re-occurred, or died in 10 years. Sheesh!

k) not really caring about the person, just the stats... having wreaked havoc on my 'Self,' which no one is measuring or recording or even asking about.

l) I guess I do not consider percentages to be my guide. I believe there is a Guide Who actually cares about my 'Self.'

m) It is hard for me to participate in a god-less world. There is nothing familiar to hold on to or sense as wholesome, good or beautiful.

n) it is so very strange to have 3 camps: the scientific people who do not recognize the God people, the scientific people do not recognize the holistic people.

What if the scientific data people actually took an interest in the God and holistic people? But, no, they can't find anything to measure, so they don't play.

o) so, the only data available is god-less, only measuring the thing they can measure.

p) the world is not really 'yes' and 'no.' there are a zillion variables.

q) it is easy to find data about TAKING the treatments, swallowing the stuff, etc... but where is the data for people who say 'no thank-you' and do not do it? Those people must exist? Do they live?

r) what if I died in 5 or 10 years with my body intact instead of tampered with by un-understandable changes, side-effects, chemical invasions, tracks of un-natural substances coursing through my veins? Foreigners, unwelcome and unable to be expelled. Irreversible damages to fill up someone's clipboard with data???

s) is the cancer gone? well, we can't be sure.

will it come back? here? someplace else related? someplace else unrelated? well, we can't be sure.

stats do not predict the future, they only read about the past.

will the treatment's side effects complicate my health? well we can't be sure.

will the treatments' side effects take my life in some other way than the cancer would have in the first place? well, we can't be sure.

t) I am ME.. I am not part of your statistics!

I remember when I decided to take anti-depressant medication, I said, "wow, now I'm a stat" because I was the age, gender and living in a place where it was common for women to fall into depression. Yet, my own story, beliefs, struggle, courage, determination, resources, path, goals, recovery, were not important to anyone.

u) I guess I am talking about losing my identity. That is a fearful thing to me. Getting swallowed up in the crowd, becoming a number so that my stats can be tallied and calculated.

v) numbers, statistics, percentages: they make it easy for someone with a clipboard to feel like they are accomplishing something, but, how is the person actually doing? who measures, cares, takes time for that? The 'nasty thing' might be 'gone' that they can measure... but that does not mean the person 'feels better' ????

w) I feel split in half: before this my life was all in one piece. I did what I believed in. My actions and my values matched. Now my body has been taken and treated with forces no one can explain, leaving my 'Self' over someplace else, no longer joined together, split off on another path... will they reconcile? reunite? separate?

~ ~ ~

My mouth moves very fast. If my words can get out before my emotions realize what's happening, maybe I won't start crying again.

"OK. That's enough," I lean back, slouched. "That is what it is like inside my head." I look up, like an animal in a trap, searching the face of the human approaching who may harm me, or may help me.

"It is all upsetting," she quietly responds. Gently. "This is where you are now. It is not the only place you have ever been, not the only place you ever will be."

"I'm stuck," I mumble, downward. I so appreciate people in the helping professions. Who would willingly approach, stay with, offer skilled help to a person in pain?

"It's hard for you to trust all of this..." She gestures to include everything cancer-related. "Can you think of another time in your life when you *did* accept medical intervention and you were glad?"

"Yes," I explained, "I tried antidepressants when I realized that I could not get out of bed. It was for the sake of my children and my husband. It was scary to swallow the pills, but I also thought of what Jesus said, 'I have come that you may have life and have it more abundantly.' Lying in bed wasn't an abundant life!"

"So, you said 'yes' to God and 'yes' to science? Is that what I heard you say?" She's pretty good at listening after all.

For a wonderful moment, I rest.

"Another time, before I had to take a scary test, another verse popped into my head." I flip back to a page near the beginning. "Here it is."

Comfort ye my people...
The voice of one crying in the wilderness:

"Prepare the way of the Lord;
Make straight in the desert
A highway for our God."
Every valley shall be exalted
And every mountain and hill brought low;
The crooked places shall be made straight
And the rough places smooth;
The glory of the Lord shall be revealed.
Isaiah 40: 1–5

"I felt like 'comfort' was something God wanted me to have. I felt like I was 'the voice crying in the wilderness,' so hopeless, so alone. But, then I felt like 'Prepare ye the way of the Lord' was meant to be my effort. That the researchers and doctors and scientists were trying to make the confusing problems and mountains of questions go from crooked and rough to become understood solutions, straight answers and smooth interventions. That I should cooperate. That in the end, the whole purpose of all the work was so that the 'glory of the Lord would be revealed.' So, I was able to take the test willingly and not force myself."

"It sounds like these Bible verses help you sort things out."

"Yes. Here are a few more." I have scribbled a few treasures in my Journal.

In my distress I called upon the Lord
and He heard my voice.
Jonah 2:2

The Lord is my strength and my shield,
In Him my heart trusts.
Psalm 28: 7

The Lord is a sun and a shield.
The Lord will give grace and glory.
No good thing will He withhold
from those who walk uprightly.
Psalm 84:11

"People help me, too. And gifts. I brought all of my 'get well' cards with me to see, and read, and feel connected to my friends." Fran's card had daisies, like our wedding. Cheryl's card made me smile with a silly joke. The ladies at church all signed a flowery card. "In-between treatments, I wear necklaces made by each of my children. See?" The little beads strung in rainbow order was made by Elise when she was about twelve. The jade pendant was from Michael for Mother's Day when he was in college. The geode came recently with a get well card from Nicholas and Johanna. When Toby was in Grade 6, he made blue and green beads on a strong string with letters spelling 'Hi' and 'Mom' on either side of a bead heart.

"Pretty special!" Her friendly face is good medicine.

"Two really special things happened when I was in Victoria," I begin to tell my story. "I had submitted my first manuscript a few days after Christmas, before I heard about this cancer diagnosis. I had already planned to go to Victoria to meet my Project Manager at the publishing company. After I found out the bad news, obviously, I realized I wouldn't be taking on too much until all of this was all over. But, I decided I would still take the ferry and go to the meeting. During the night, in my hotel, a word arrived. 'Tranquility.' The next day, walking with a friend, browsing in the gift stores, I noticed a tiny, golden angel. 'Tranquility' seemed to be her message. I brought that tiny golden angel with me. She helps me sleep. In fact, I think I will go look at her right now."

I return my empty tea cup. Fold the afghan. Turn to go. "Thank-you for listening!"

"Any time. Good night."

~ ~ ~

Daylight. I must have slept. Yes, I did. I remember my dream.

Three people were bowed in prayer outside the door of an institution. I heard a man's voice.

"Heavenly Father we know that you said, 'Where two or three are gathered together in my name, there am I in the midst of them.' And 'Whatever you ask in my name, it will be done for you by my Father who is in heaven.' Today, we ask you for Tranquility and peace of mind for Eleanor so she can rest, trust, sleep."

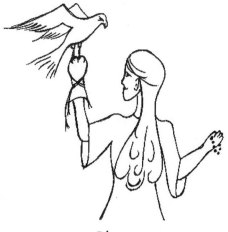

Chapter 8
Tuesday, April 21, 2015
The Missing Piece
The Missing Peace

I think it's kind of interesting the way things get to be
the way the people work with their machines.
Serenity's a long time coming to me
in fact I don't believe I know what it means any more.
—*Eclipse, performed by John Denver*[25]

~ ~ ~

Tuesday. Wednesday. Thursday.
Tuesday. Wednesday. Thursday.
I speak in rhythm as I stride along the sidewalk on my way
to morning Mass.
That's 20 seconds – times both sides – is 40 seconds – times 3
sessions – equals 120 seconds – divided by 60 seconds – equals

– 2 minutes! Only two minutes left! Then I will be free! No more radiation. Free!

Only three more sleeps. Only three more apples. Only six more muffins. Only two more minutes.

I think I'll make it!

My eyes drink in every tulip, open and bright. I breathe in the lilac scent, abundant and bowing down. I notice a cute cottage. I admire the stonework along a path. Everything seems bold and clear and good this morning.

It started with the Psalm I read in the Prayer Book when I first woke up.

> They go out, they go out full of tears
> carrying seed for the sowing.
> They come back, they come back full of song
> carrying their sheaves.
> Psalm 126: 5-6

That would be me!

I slide into my place in the little chapel and open my book to the right page. I glance a silent greeting to the others.

Loretta always mentions people by name who are ill when she prays. She offered to pray for me, too. I have never heard my name spoken so tenderly before. She comes early and stays late. Prayer book before Mass. Rosary after Mass. Every morning.

Robert sits to my left. He gave me a ride last week when my radiation appointment was too close to the end of Mass. I didn't want to miss Mass!

Moses! I've never met anyone named Moses! He just told me his name last week. Each time I have 'held up my arm to prevail against the enemy' like the story of Moses in Exodus, I didn't know that I also had a smile from a man named Moses before Mass in the morning.

The leader enters in his white robe. Sylvester has been the Deacon here, teaching us how to sing many parts of the daily prayers. He is a young man from Africa. Last week he was ordained a priest!

~ ~ ~

One week ago, the church was packed full for the Sacrament of Holy Orders. The choir was accompanied by musicians on guitar, cello, violin, flute and piano. The ritual began with the dramatic procession of the Knights of Columbus wearing their colourful sashes, flowing capes, white gloves and plumed hats. I counted. There were 34 priests, seminarians, deacons and the bishop on the chancel.

I have been to the Sacraments of Baptism, Reconciliation, Holy Communion, Confirmation and a Wedding. I have also attended a few Catholic funerals. This was the first time I have attended an Ordination.

The choir led the opening hymn. It was based on the same Psalm that Kevin and I had printed on our engagement announcements.

One thing I have I desired of the Lord,
that will I seek after,
that I may dwell in the house of the Lord
all the days of my life,
to behold the beauty of the Lord
and to inquire in His temple.
Psalm 27

The Mass proceeded. After the Scripture readings, the congregation recited the Nicean Creed.

And at that moment, for me, it was as if time stood still.

> I believe in one God, the Father almighty,
> maker of heaven and earth,
> of all things visible and invisible.
>> *Nicene Creed*

How many times have I said it?
Look! Listen!
The answer to my question is right there!
The missing piece!
What are some of the invisible things God created? My mind raced for answers. Magnetism. Gravity. Electricity. Invisible forces. Mysterious. Harnessed. Useful. Yes, Radiation! We can't see them, but God made them. We can use them for harm or for good.

The ritual proceeded. Each part meaningful. Words and actions combined in this sacred rite. Surely, God poured blessings on everyone present.

Surely, it all made a very personal impression on me.

~ ~ ~

This morning is the first time I have been present when this new priest officiates at the Mass. Now he is authorized to consecrate the Host to prepare for Holy Communion.

Again, time stands still. I hear familiar words as if for the first time.

As he blesses the bread and then the wine, the priest always says,

> Blessed are you, Lord God of all creation,
> for through your goodness we have received
> the bread we offer you
> fruit of the earth and work of human hands...
>> —*Prayer at the altar*

That's it!
Another missing piece!
How could I have missed it? It's all the same!
Everything we use: table, chair, cup, spoon, clothing, shoes, paper, pencil. They all come from the earth *and* the work of human hands.
Science? Inventions? Medicine? It is all the same.
I have been so confused, agonizing, really. Now, it is as clear as day. It is so obvious, now that I see it.
Relief. Cleansed. Balanced. Renewed.
Grateful.
The missing peace is restored.

∾ ∾ ∾

The Falcon soars, dives, snatches another eel.

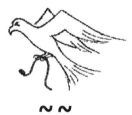

∾ ∾

Only two more left!

∾ ∾

But, there's more.
The evening prayer book shares this Psalm.

I sought the Lord, and He answered me,
and delivered me from all my fears.
Look to Him and be radiant.
Psalm 34: 4–5

How can the Lord do that?
Bring me to the right place at the right time?
Open my eyes, ears, heart.
Shine with His radiance!
Show me the missing piece.
Give me the missing peace.

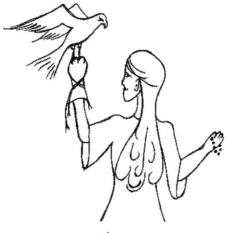

Chapter 9
Thursday, April 23, 2015
Last Day

I am the eagle I live in high country
in rocky cathedrals that reach to the sky.
I am the hawk and there's blood on my feathers
but time it still turning they soon will be dry.
And all those who see me and all who believe in me
share in the freedom I feel when I fly.
—*The Eagle and the Hawk, performed by John Denver*[26]

~

7:00
It's my last day!

Awake, dressed and out.

I walk briskly. Up a few blocks. Over a few blocks. I like to take a slightly different route each time, past apartment buildings or a playground, stores or a church, houses with modern geometric lines or charming cottages. I have never lived in a city. There is lots to see. The gardens look lovely with golden daffodils, and bright orange tulips, and pale pink blossoms opening on flowering trees. The forsythia is bursting yellow everywhere. I can smell the hyacinths. The lilacs have opened, too.

As always, I carry a shoulder bag with food, water bottle, prayer book, notebook and a place to stow my sweater when the sun warms the day. Walking while munching on the bran muffins and the apple I brought from home, I feel like shouting to the sky, "It's my last day!"

~

The prayer time begins at 7:30.

It seems like every word has been perfectly placed for my own personal encouragement.

Inspired by the text, my heart provides additional messages in-between the lines.

Lord, as daylight fills the sky,
May our lives mirror our love for You,
whose wisdom has brought us into being
and whose care guides us on our way.

(That is exactly how I felt while walking to church this morning.)

You do not allow us to be tested beyond our ability.
Strengthen the weak and raise up the fallen.

(Yes, indeed, I have been tested. I have made it through! He is the One who strengthened me. By myself, I would have fallen and remained in despair.)

The reading today is from Psalm 99.

The Lord is King...
He is supreme over all...
Among His priests were
Aaron and Moses... and Samuel

(Aaron and Moses have helped me since that first day when I recognized that like them, I needed to keep my arms up in order to win the battle.) (Samuel is a name I gave my husband long ago because it means 'asked of God.')

They called on the Lord and He answered.
To them He spoke in the pillar of cloud...

(How is this possible? I called on the Lord that first scary night in the motel, and He answered and comforted me, with these very same names and ideas that are right here in the prayers on my last day. I feel safe now, protected and provided for.)
Next is a description of Jesus I have never heard before:

You were willing to live as a stranger in our world.
Be mindful of those
who are separated from family and homeland.

(like me)

After all of my anxiety about the radiation treatment, here is the same word used to describe God for the purpose of healing those who face death.

All powerful and ever-living God,
shine with the light of Your radiance
on the people who live in the shadow of death.

And, now that I will be returning to my usual volunteer activities and preparing lessons for the children at church, I hear this prayer:

At the beginning of this day,
fill us with zeal for serving You.
Good Shepherd,
please give your leaders unfailing faith,
lively hope, loving concern,
and help them to be an instrument
nourished by Your Grace
to bring Your children back to You.

And the closing prayer to read this evening:

Lord, we thank you for guiding us
through the course of this days work.
In your compassion forgive
the sins we have committed through human weakness.
We ask this through our Lord Jesus Christ, Your Son...
(radiant with love and mercy, truth and wisdom,
compassion and kindness)
...who lives and reigns with the Father...
(Almighty, creator of things visible and invisible)
...and the Holy Spirit ...
(Counsellor, Comforter, Guide)
...One God forever and ever. AMEN

~

8:00
Mass

So sweet. So familiar. So nourishing. I may never be in this place again, or see these people again, but we are forever connected as 'Brothers and Sisters in the Christ.'

∼

10:00

It is not too far to walk to Inspire Health. There is a yoga session this morning. It helps me so much to be out of the scientific, mathematical, data-driven realm and be here with others who share a softer view of life, bodies, health, the planet, people who are willing to explore complementary ways to participate in one's own health.

It's a quiet hour, calming, listening to instructions, following the moves and postures, becoming self-aware. How differently I feel. On the table during the radiation treatment, I am stiff, tight, forcing myself. Trying not to feel any physical sensations. Shushing my inner thoughts. Here, I stretch and enjoy the physical sensations of my own muscles and joints, breath and heart beat. I trust the leader and open to her voice and guidance. I become aware of inner pathways and new ideas emerge.

I have to leave right away and walk fast to get back for my very last counselling appointment!

∼

11:30

"This is the one thing I will be sad to leave." I smile at Ruth. "Thank-you for coming with me to the appointment with Dr. O last week. It was so helpful. When I am emotional or stressed, it is hard to get up the courage to ask questions, hear the answers, and stand up for myself if I don't understand. It's hard to remember what he says. Having you there was calming and kept me focused. I felt confident and safe. I had an extra pair of eyes and ears to help me remember what happened and interpret what was meant."

"I was so glad to be invited," Ruth replied, "I have never attended a session. I coach so many people without actually participating in their experience. It was fascinating to see the diagram of your body and the treatment plan map and see how the radiation would pass through the breast and chest on the diagonal."

"Do you see why I was so frightened? I thought the whole thing went straight down through my whole left side! Only after I found a diagram on the internet did I see the diagonal and how carefully they actually avoid as much as they can while targeting the breast. But, the chest is rounded and the rays are straight, so there is a skim across the lung and heart." It is such a relief to be able to speak in a straightforward way with someone. I don't have to shelter her from alarming information, or erupting emotions, or be 'polite,' or skirt controversial topics.

Re-tracing our time together I continue. "You were very brave to come into the radiation treatment room with me for that one appointment, too. You could see all of the equipment and preparation for the procedure and have an idea what each patient has to undergo."

"I have had a tour of the treatment rooms, but it is different to go in with a real person who you care about," Ruth observes.

"And I still have six months that I can contact you?" I lean forward on my chair, searching her face.

"Yes, if it is cancer related. We can phone, e-mail, or you can come in."

I am so glad. I can't really be sure how I will feel when I go home. Relieved, but you never know when emotions come unexpectedly like a powerful wave or swirling storm.

"Remember when I first came in... all red faced and alarmed and crying. I actually don't remember anything I said that day, only that you were looking into my eyes and I felt safe. No matter how confused I was, you were going to be steady and not get mad at me or try to talk me out of my feelings." I chuckle, "I know I am a very fast talker! You are a very fast listener!"

Her eyes are like an oasis. Safe. Calm. Welcoming. Refreshing.

It seems important to me to summarize from the very beginning. "When we spoke on the phone during the month before treatments, I told you that I had a double plan. Do you remember?"

"Yes!" Ruth's smile lights up. "You were going to bring five disguises and sign up for a counselling appointment every single day!"

"Yes! I could not possibly imagine making it through without talking to you for an hour after each treatment!"

"And you had decided to pretend that you were in a science fiction movie." She has a very good memory.

I'm glad my imagination could provide something humorous. It was a lot better than the scenes that my dire fears constructed.

"How did the visualization of the falcon and the marsh help you through it all?" It is amazing to me that she can recall my details when she has so many clients moving through her office.

"That was one thing I focused on every day and sometimes all night. The position I had to hold with my left arm up was the same posture as a falconer. While the technicians got ready, left me alone in the room, and the treatment proceeded, I gave myself a full experience in my imagination. This visualization kept me calm and gave me a way to agree with the prescribed treatment, even though it seemed so foreign to anything I have ever anticipated participating in."

Gesturing to demonstrate, I continued describing the scene. "Today, the last of the adult eels will all be removed. This is how

I have imagined the cancer cells, which have contaminated my body and how they are all being destroyed. The next part of my treatment will begin in two weeks. I have to swallow a pill every day for five years to block any place there might be one-more-cell. It is so creepy to think that there might be any cancer cells that can wait up to five years to grow big enough to be discovered! So, I have another part of the visualization to encourage myself to follow through with it." Ruth is listening intently to my descriptions. "Now a chalky white tablet will be dissolved into the water and any remaining eggs the eels have laid will be destroyed, without damaging the insect, fish, bird, or mammal populations who depend on the marsh." It is all so clear in my mind.

Ruth's face shows me that she appreciates the difficulty I have faced, the challenges and obstacles I overcame. There is much to be happy about today.

"I am so glad I got to meet your husband," she continues our review. "Kevin came to your appointment during that first week. And later your Mother and Papa Joe."

"Yes, and I am so glad they know you, so they know who I am talking about." I pause to form words around a new idea. "I just realized. That is another whole layer of this experience. None of my friends or family know what it is like here. Nobody here knows me at home. I hardly want to describe every little thing. So, all anyone can say is, 'How are you doing?' and all I can say is, 'OK.' That is not very satisfying!"

"What are your plans for the rest of today? For tomorrow? When you get home?" Ruth knows how much it helps me stay oriented and out of depressing thoughts to focus on the near future and action steps I plan to take.

"I have decided to stay for one day after the treatments are over. I have an appointment tomorrow at the laser clinic to have the two ink dots they call tattoos removed! So, I will go to Mass, another yoga session at Inspire Health, then go down to get the ink zapped away. It takes almost an hour to walk that far. But I will be back in time to take the bus back to where my husband will meet me! One last time!"

I can see on her face a look of anticipation. "I seem to remember you talking about something else?"

"Yes! I am going to throw away all of my clothes! Shoes! Socks! PJs. Everything! I don't want to bring home any Kooties."

"What are you going to wear home?"

"I don't know yet! I will have time tomorrow to go shopping. I intend to find a graduation dress to wear home! I have been looking in all the stores. White cotton summer gowns. Hippy tie-dye wrap skirts. Elegant fabrics from India. I've been to classy ladies wear stores. I strolled through the mall. I even went into a few Thrift Stores so I would know what there is to choose from. I know I'll find the perfect dress!"

"Now," I reach into my bag, "I have presents for you. One from Kevin and one from me."

Surprised, carefully, enjoying the moment, Ruth unwraps the wooden box Kevin made. It has a lid and a small hollow space for coins, keys or other special items. After I explain how Kevin made it, she admires a small Fairy Doll I made from a flexible pipe-cleaner and autumn coloured silk flower petals for the dress and hat, wings and boots.

The clock says it is time for me to go.

Saying "Good-bye" doesn't feel final, now that she has a visual reminder of our time together.

~

By the time I walk back to the dormitory, the lunch hour is half way over. I'm glad. I don't care what is left for me to eat. I don't intend to make any conversation. I find an empty table to sip my soup and eat my sandwich.

~

1:00

Time for my next appointment.

It is that old familiar feeling of being back on the conveyor belt.

There is one more important decision to make. I have been assigned to see Dr. P, who I have never seen before and I will never see again.

I silence the echo spoken by people who want to take the 'Natural' route. They call standard forms of cancer treatment: 'Cut. Burn. Poison.'

I've had the surgery. I've had the radiation. Now I will learn about the medication that is intended to snuff out any remaining cancer cells.

I am not sure where to go, so I ask at the nurses' station. Upstairs I meet in a small office with Dr. P to learn about the medication that is recommended. What a long list of possible side effects! What a long time I have to swallow this chemical! Every day for five years!

She explains everything clearly. "The cancer cells want estrogen. The cells absorb this medication instead. It blocks the estrogen. The cells die." I wonder what other functions estrogen has in my body? I wonder why five years is the magic number? I wonder what this chemical is, and where it is made, and what is costs, and why it is free in Canada, and where I will get enough to last for five years? I imagine the mountain of pills that are manufactured, the truck loads being delivered, the millions of women who swallow it. But I don't really care. It is my last day and I have very little curiosity and no resistance left. Besides, I decided early on that I was going to do this. I was convinced when my husband's friend, Fred, told me, "My wife had the surgery but said 'No' to the radiation and medication. In five years the cancer came back and she died."

I certainly do think it is possible for there to be 'one cell' lurking somewhere in the breast after the disturbance caused by the biopsy, by the surgery, and perhaps other microscopic beginnings that cannot be observed yet with the mammogram. I agreed to take the radiation to destroy any cancer cells in the immediate area.

I hate to imagine, but, it is possible that one cell has escaped and moved into other parts of the body. It would be much harder to discover. This particular kind of breast cancer cell can also form a tumour in the bone, liver, lung or brain! Dreadful thought! Yes, I will take the medication. It will travel throughout my whole body, seeking any tiny sneaky, stubborn, cells dormant or lurking, plotting my demise, silently waiting to re-populate a new colony. But, no! I will snuff them out before they can begin!

There are rumours that this medication can cause weight gain. Eight to twenty pounds! That won't be fun! There are rumours that you get more and stronger hot flashes. Also not much fun! However, these are minor possibilities compared with the disastrous recurrence of a cancer colony beginning again.

I have no hesitation after Dr. P tells me that this medication has been used since the 1970s with many long-term studies and follow-up data collected. I will do as instructed.

She prints my prescription and gives me directions to the pharmacy in a distant part of the building to get the first round of pills. After this, I will need to travel to a hospital closer to home to pick up 90 days of pills at a time. More days away from home. More gas money. Yet, a small price to pay for peace of mind.

~

Back down the stairs. Through the familiar halls. Sign in with the bar code ID card. Sit in familiar waiting room.

2:20

My name is called. Only 40 seconds left. Then I'm done.

I quit using the hospital gown a long time ago. I simply zip off my sweat shirt, toss it on the chair and step to the centre of the room to lie on the table. The green light cross-hairs meet at the ink dot target. My left arm goes up. My right hand clutches the eagle pendant and the ten purple beads. This keeps me focused on the world of Nature and the world of Faith. In both ways God has provided for me from the start.

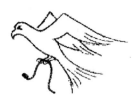

Instead of counting the 20 seconds on each side, today I have decided to count down from 40! When I get to zero: I will be D-O-N-E!

Click. Hum. 40-39-38-37... Click.

The machine moves from my upper right to the second angle at my lower left.

Click. Hum. 7-6-5-4-3-2-1 Click.

I get out of there as fast as I can.

Although I do not have a full range of motion on my left side, I stretch and breathe deeply in silent celebration for a few minutes in the fresh air and sunshine.

Then back into the hallways for one last appointment.

3:10

Dr. O, the radiologist has moved way. I knew that he would not be present at the end of my treatment when I agreed to be under his care. Now it is the last day, and I have to meet yet another doctor I have never seen before and I will never see again.

'The Doctor of the week' happens to be Dr. Q.

He wants to know whether the 'sunburn' was severe.

"No. Do you want to see my nipple?"

Awkward.

"Not necessary."

Good thing. I am so nearly finished. I don't have much stamina left for exposure.

I want to know if I can have the doctor with the laser remove the ink dots tomorrow.

"No. You don't want to add any more stress to the body's healing process. Wait a month."

Disappointing.

"Do you have anything to say about your over-all experience here?" He's holding a clipboard, pen poised, just like all the others.

"I found it hard to communicate with Dr. O, the radiologist. He was very scientific, but he was always surprised when I showed any emotion. Hey! This is making a pretty big impact on my life!"

"Yes," Dr. Q shares a glimpse behind the scenes. "When Dr. O gave presentations, all the doctors learned a lot, but he doesn't have a very warm 'bedside manner.' Several others have noticed."

"Can I throw this away now?" I am eager to tear up my ID card.

"You betcha! The whole reason you did this is so that you'll never need it again!"

Done!

So, I now have to go to make a phone call to cancel my appointment tomorrow with Dr. R, the laser doctor, and re-book for some time in late May. Oh! I am so disappointed!

Look at the time! I've missed the bus! And now I have no reason to stay tomorrow.

Here's a puzzle to solve. What to do for an extra day in a place you don't want to be?

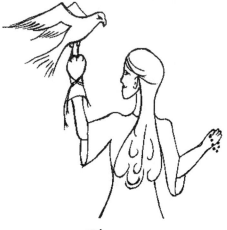

Chapter 10
Friday, April 24, 2015
Exit

Country roads take me home to the place I belong!
—*Country Roads,* performed by John Denver[27]

I notice an uncomfortable mixture of disappointment and anticipation today.

Maybe there will be important details at some time during this day? After all: it is not what I planned. Yet, God knew that Dr. Q would say 'No' about the laser, and what time my appointments were scheduled, and that I would miss the bus, and that I would have no appointments today. So? Maybe He has a little something planned for me, like a scavenger hunt? Maybe there is treasure hiding that I can see, now that I do not have my usual routines? What can I find just around the corner?

I am curious.

I am alert.

As usual, I wake early, reach for the clothing and the shoulder bag I prepared last night, step into the washroom, and then quietly move down the hallway.

I go to the library with the comfy couches and lakeside scene from the patio. I have privacy. It feels like a cocoon.

Opening my thick, red Prayer Book brings a sense of belonging. Tradition links me with millions of priests, deacons, monks, nuns and laity around the world who will read this page today gathered in churches, monasteries, convents and individually in private homes. Perhaps thousands will be reading the Liturgy of the Hours right now, in my time zone.

I have kept a fairly consistent habit of reading this book for five years. There are yellow, purple, green, white and blue ribbons to mark the hymns, morning, daytime and evening prayers and Sunday readings. I have never made marks, underlines or notes in the margin... until now.

At daybreak, be merciful to me.
Make known to me the path I must walk.

"This was my first thought. So many have walked this path." I wrote in the margin when I was first diagnosed.

This prayer:

You created us as a sign of Your power
and elected us Your people to show Your goodness.

This reading:

Therefore I am content with weakness,
with mistreatment, with distress,
with persecutions and difficulties

for the sake of Christ;
for when I am powerless,
it is then that I am strong.
2 Corinthians 12:10

Both are a little confusing. As a new Catholic, I am still not entirely used to the attitude towards suffering. Most people want to avoid suffering. Suffering often shakes a person's faith. 'Why did God let this happen?' A person might be tempted to move away from anything related to God or the church.

But, Catholics see it as a way to be near Jesus, to be like Him, to participate with Him who suffered in our place, in some way to take on a small part of His suffering, to realize that while suffering He was able to forgive, to realize the ways we have hurt others, to say 'Yes' to the gift of His forgiveness, to learn mercy from the experience.

My brothers, count it as pure joy
when you are involved in every sort of trial.
Realize that when your faith is tested
this makes for endurance.
Let endurance come to its perfection
so that you may be fully mature and lacking in nothing.
James 1:2–4

Well! I certainly have been tested! I certainly have strengthened my endurance! I'm not sure that I can count it as pure joy? Perhaps I have yet to become 'fully mature.' Maybe there is something I cannot foresee up ahead?

Closing prayer:

Father all powerful,
let Your radiance dawn in our lives
that we may walk in the light of Your law
with You as our leader.

There's that word, 'radiance', again! Only this time, I want to open my heart, and calm my anxiety, and flow with trust, and allow myself to relax, and accept this day, this circumstance, knowing that I can walk forward with confidence knowing that He is the Leader.

It's my last muffin-and-apple walk to Mass.

I don't feel so much that I am 'getting away from' something today. I feel more like 'I have chosen to go towards' something today. I am not forcing my feet to take another step, watching the clock, deliberately arriving at appointments, clamping my jaw, clenching my fists, keeping my emotions shut down.

Today everything is optional. Except for getting to the bus, I don't have to be at a certain place at a certain time. What will I choose to do? What will I move towards? What will I turn away from?

I choose to let down my guard, take down the walls I have been protecting myself with, allow for the possibility that goodness with flow to me. I choose to turn my face up to the sky, to notice the birds, to admire the gardens, to enjoy my own stride, to stand tall and breathe deep. I choose to enter the church with a sense of wonder, to let my eyes and my heart fill with the beauty of the flowers, candles, figurines, paintings, colourful glass. I choose to open my ears and heart, and savour the reading of Scripture, repetition of the prayers, join in the hymns and responses.

Instead of a life raft to cling to in a deadly storm, it feels like a banquet today, generous, soothing. I appreciate every part of my 'Self.' Heart, Spirit, Mind, Body are each nourished.

I greet the people I have met, letting them know I will be leaving today, letting them know that I appreciate their kind welcome and encouraging prayers.

My friends have signed a card. It is my favourite prayer.

God has created me
to do him some definite service;
He has committed some work to me
which He has not committed to another.
I have my mission -
I may never know what it is in this life,
but I shall be told of it in the next.

I am a link in a chain,
a bond of connection between persons.
He has not created me for naught,
I shall do good,
I shall do his work.
I shall be an angel of peace,
a preacher of truth
in my own place
while not intending it -
if I do but keep
His Commandments.

Therefore, I will trust Him.
Whatever, wherever I am,
I can never be thrown away.

If I am in sickness,
my sickness may serve Him;
in perplexity,
my perplexity may serve Him;
if I am in sorrow,
my sorrow may serve Him.
He does nothing in vain.
He knows what He is about.
He may take away my friends.
He may throw me among strangers.
He may make me feel desolate,
make my spirits sink,
hide my future from me -
still He knows what He is about.
              Prayer of Cardinal J. H. Newman

I wrote in my day-book that there is an exercise session at Inspire Health. It would be fun to drop in. But first, there's a dress shop nearby that I want to explore. I haven't found my 'graduation dress' yet!

"How can I help you?" the sales lady eagerly approaches.

"I have been admiring your selection for a few weeks. Today I hope to make a decision," I let her know I am in earnest. I browse the springtime pastels, the airy blouses, the scarves and accessories, the glittery belts and bags. I'm looking for something that will help me remember that 'I am Me.' I am not an office employee or business entrepreneur. I am not a shapely young fashion diva. I am not a sporty fitness gal. But, I'm not an old lady, either. Do they make clothes for me?

Although they attract my eye, I don't think one of those white lacy gowns would last a minute at home. I buy warm clothes and clothes for working in the garden at Thrift Stores. I don't have to impress anyone or show up at an event. Today, the price tag doesn't matter (too much). This is for 'Me.' A strange, rare experience!

I turn this way and that in the fitting room, returning a few, keeping a few.

"This is what I am looking for." I show her a gauzy, sleeveless, royal blue tunic with a trendy, long asymmetrical hemline. Soft grey pussy-willows signal the 'Back-to-Nature' look I am seeking. "But I need sleeves," I explain, "and leggings." My home in the mountains is rarely warm enough for me to enjoy such a summery frock.

It is easy to locate a royal blue tee-shirt with three-quarter length sleeves. As a bonus, it is made with a new kind of bamboo fabric. Black leggings are also readily available.

Across the hall, a pair of black sandals caught my eye.

I feel simply buoyant as I pay for my selections.

11:00

My Day-Book says, 'Relax and Visualize at Inspire Health,' so up the stairs I go, entering the little mirrored gym.

I take my place on the wooden floor with a yoga mat, cushion and blanket. 'Guided Imagery' is enjoyable to me. The leader sets up tea-light candles, soft music, dims the lights and invites participants to rest and become still. She tells a comforting story filled with scenes of Nature and peaceful observations.

Becoming aware of sensations within my own body helps me find and let loose the tense muscles, which have held so much resistance for so many days and nights. No longer constricted, my lungs and limbs stretch and take their rightful space.

The narrator takes us to a high plateau. From there we can look down at the beautiful Earth, see our own Life Path and become grateful for the people who have encouraged us along the way.

In the quiet, I look for ways that Air, Earth, Fire and Water have nourished and strengthened me. I wonder which of my friends has shared these qualities with me?

Air. As my lungs expand, music comes to mind. Singing. Playing an instrument. Being part of a choir or band. In and out, the air moves. Some friends come and go, but each shares their song. My smile flickers each time a musical friend comes into the scene. Creativity. Team spirit. Traditions.

Earth. I recall my first counsellor, who taught me how to 'be grounded.' At this moment, here, now, the world does not seem to be a whirling tornado or dangerous roller coaster. I don't need to hold on for dear life. I can allow the earth to hold and cradle me. Stability. Abundance. Trust.

Fire. Man's best friend. Man's worst enemy. Emotions, like fire, can rampage out of control. It has taken a great deal of effort for me to rein in my emotions. But, fire can also be life-giving, warmth can be soothing, light can be guiding. Ruth has certainly helped me tend the fire, naming emotions, allowing expression, guiding towards resolution, instead of being afraid, or ashamed, or confused by my own process. Safety. Clarity. Comfort.

Water. Flowing, pooling, rising, raining, always moving in a cycle, necessary for life, a symbol of forgiveness and renewal, able to take new shapes, a force for action. I am usually rigid. I value friends who adapt and adjust, who offer alternatives and can make changes gently. Cleansing. Satisfying. Ever-changing.

Each element and each friend leaves an imprint in my imagination to treasure.

The narrator brings us down the slope and suggests we meet face-to-face with someone who was especially trustworthy and kind.

Grammie! I feel safe and protected when I am with Grammie! Tears form and spill as, in my imagination, I run to her. "Grammie! Grammie! Keep me safe! I'm scared! Hold me tight!"

The leader of our session is moving to each participant with soft footsteps, covering each with a blanket, placing a soothing eye-bag, offering a warm, firm touch. The session is almost over.

"You OK?" she whispers as she gives my shoulders a kind, encouraging touch.

"My Grammie loves me," I can barely whisper. My Grandmother's little daughter died. I am named after that child. A mother endured the loss of an innocent child. I have experienced the loss of my own innocence. I feel connected to Grammie now. Now I know a little of the powerless feeling, yet the personal formation of faith that grows from the experience of Grief.

With no intent to draw attention to myself, other participants offer a hug or kind smile as they leave.

One young woman brings me a box of tissues and stays to offer a listening ear.

"Grammie took care of me when I was an infant. She read aloud, recited poems, taught me Bible stories and songs. She held my hand while I crossed the scary log bridge. To me, she is like the Guardian Angel in the painting."

I am astonished. I have offered not one word of comfort to anyone the whole time I have been here. This woman, perhaps twenty years younger than me, introduced herself at a previous session. "I'm Lisa. I was diagnosed the Stage 4 breast cancer. It's in my liver now." How can she give? How can she smile? Isn't liver cancer terminal?

Calm now, I move towards the door, "I have to get back to the lodge. I have to catch the bus."

"Let me give you a ride." Lisa's generous chocolate eyes are so nourishing, comforting, strengthening.

"Really? It's more than a two-hour drive!"

"I'll phone my husband. He'll say yes. We do stuff like this all the time!"

I have one more quick errand. There was another dress downstairs that has an aqua blue fabric that reminded me of Grammie's church dress. I am going to buy it, too.

It's Friday and the dormitory is nearly empty already.

Quickly, I phone Kevin to tell him to meet me earlier than expected. Quickly, my bags are packed. Quickly, I change into my graduation outfit.

Tied in a bundle, I shove the clothing I have been wearing during these treatments into the garbage can, shoes and all!

There's only one thing left to do.

I cross the parking lot, enter the dreaded hallways one last time. I march to the receptionist's desk.

"Bubbles, Please!" I grin. "It's my last day!"

Even the quilts on the wall look more cheery.

It is infinitely more pleasant to travel with people you want to talk to. It is infinitely more pleasant to travel towards home!

Lisa and her husband, Scott, describe their favourite volunteer project. "We buy gift cards at grocery stores and coffee shops and give them to homeless people." They offer me the use of their tent trailer if I ever want to come for a visit or tour the area.

They have taken their children to Disneyland, the Maritimes, they go camping, and hunt for treasure with a metal detector, and geo-cache. Lisa confides in me, telling me about her security item. She gets a sense of hope and renewal when a ladybug lands on or near her.

In a flash, I realize that they have given me enough information for me to make a 'Talking Quilt'[28] as a thank-you for this day together.

I said at the start that I never wanted to help anyone.

Now I have been helped by a person who knows she has a life-threatening form of cancer. Her example gives me an entirely new perspective on everything.

Kevin is at the parking lot to meet me. For two-and-a-half hours we laugh and talk and I blare the John Denver music.

I want to live.
I want to grow.
I want to see.
I want to know.
I want to share
what I can give.
I want to be.
I want to live!
    —John Denver[29]

Wrapped in each other's arms, my husband whispers his heartfelt private thoughts.

"I didn't know what you would need," Kevin's voice quavers. Is that a tear in his eye? "I was ready to help you get dressed, wash your hair, do all the lifting, and sweeping, and washing." He never told me he was so alarmed. "I'm so glad you are home. Safe. Thank-you for giving me You."

Twonight we celebrate a sweet homecoming.

If you enjoyed
10 Days in April
...a detour through breast cancer
watch for future titles Eleanor Deckert is working on

10 Days in May... plant a seed and watch it grow

10 Days in June... one thousand dollars

10 Days in July... first fruits

10 Days in August... so many good-byes

10 Days in September... learning... teaching

10 Days in October... glad, sad, mad, afraid and thanksgiving

10 Days in November... maiden, mother, widow

Titles currently available through the Author's web page

www.eleanordeckert.com
also at Chapters/Indigo Bookstores

or order on-line from the publisher
books.friesenpress.com/store

Book 1 ~ 10 Days in December... where dreams meet reality

Book 2 ~ 10 Days in January... 1 Husband...
2 Brothers... 3 Sons... 4 Dads

Book 3 ~ 10 Days in February... Limitations

Book 4 ~ 10 Days in March... Possibilities

Book 3 & Book 4 in one volume

Book 5 ~ 10 Days in April... a detour through breast cancer

Endnotes

1   Song Writer: John Denver Follow Me. Publisher: Sony/ATV Music Publishing LLC, Warner/Chappell Music, Inc., Reservoir One Music, Resevoir Media Management Inc., BMG Rights Management US, LLC

2   Songwriter: John DenverPoems, Prayers And Promises lyrics © Warner/Chappell Music, Inc., Kobalt Music Publishing Ltd.

3   The story of Nicholas' birth is recorded in Chapter 4, Book 4, '10 Days in February... Limitations Book 3 & 10 Days in March... Possibilities' © 2018 by, Eleanor Deckert published by FreisenPress.

4   Songwriter: John Denver For Baby lyrics © Reservoir Media Management INC, BMG Rights Management US, LLC

5   A description of this sad day is recorded in Book 2, '10 Days in January... 1 Husband... 2 Brothers... 3 Sons... 4 Dads' © 2016 by, Eleanor Deckert published by FreisenPress.

6   This fear of 'insanity' and frightening, invisible, powerful medical treatments is woven throughout my life and mentioned in both Book 1 '10 Days in December... where dreams meet reality' and Book 2 '10 Days in January... 1 Husband... 2 Brothers... 3 Sons... 4 Dads' © 2016 by, Eleanor Deckert published by FreisenPress.

7   Words and music by John Denver, What One Man Can Do lyrics © Reservoir Media Management INC

8   On December 28th, to mark the anniversary of that first frigid -40°C day, I had completed my first manuscript and sent it in. Five days later, I learned that I had breast cancer! The first 10 days that we lived in our 'Back-to-the-Land' log cabin is described in Book 1, '10 Days in December... where dreams meet reality' © 2016 by, Eleanor Deckert published by FreisenPress.

9   Search on-line for Clearwater Times, Valley Voices, Eleanor Deckert

10 Search on-line for Eleanor Deckert, Valley Sentinel, Valemount, BC: topics of articles: Second Hand, Gifts, Learn from Others, Do It Yourself, Free, Belong to a Group, Do Without, What do I Really Need, Keep the family together, Share an Experience, Family Traditions, Steady Income, Volunteer, Bartering

11 Fran and her husband Archie, were the first to welcome us into their family when we arrived as young newly-weds in 1978. Described in Book 1: How we met. How they helped us find land and build the cabin. Our first Christmas together. '10 Days in December... where dreams meet reality' © 2016 by, Eleanor Deckert published by FreisenPress.

12 I invented 'Talking Quilts' as an educational 'toy' to encourage language development. Alternating denim and picture squares of fabric all relating to a theme stimulate story telling, learning, questions and pretend. See photos on author's web page www.eleanordeckert.com '10 Days in April... detour through breast cancer' Book 5, Chapter 3. by, Eleanor Deckert © 2018 published by FreisenPress.

13 '10 Days in January... 1 Husband... 2 Brothers... 3 Sons.. 4 Dads' © 2016 Eleanor Deckert, published by FreisenPress Chapter 3... describes the day when my Daddy died.

14 Seasons in the Sun, recorded in the 1970s by Terry Jacks, re-written from Jacques Brel

15 Cat's in the Cradle by Harry Chapin

16 Songwriters: John Denver, Michael C Taylor, Richard L Dick Kniss Sunshine On My Shoulders lyrics © Warner/Chappell Music, Inc., Reservoir One Music, Kobalt Music Publishing Ltd., Reservoir Media Management INC, BMG Rights Management US,

17 Songwriters: John Denver, Michael C Taylor, Richard L Dick Kniss Sunshine On My Shoulders lyrics © Warner/Chappell Music, Inc., Reservoir One Music, Kobalt Music Publishing Ltd., Reservoir Media Management INC, BMG Rights Management US, LLC

18   Songwriter: John Denver Looking For Space lyrics © Warner/Chappell Music, Inc., Kobalt Music Publishing Ltd.

19   Exodus 13: 21

20   Songwriter: John Denver For Baby lyrics © Reservoir Media Management INC, BMG Rights Management US, LLC

21   The development of my relationship with Papa Joe is recorded in Chapter 3 of Book 2, '10 Days in January... 1 Husband... 2 Brothers... 3 Sons.. 4 Dads' © 2016 Eleanor Deckert, published by FreisenPress see web page for photos www.eleanordeckert.com

22   '10 Days in December... where dreams meet reality' © 2016 by, Eleanor Deckert published by FreisenPress.

23   Songwriter: John Denver Poems, Prayers And Promises lyrics © Warner/Chappell Music, Inc., Kobalt Music Publishing Ltd.

24   More about Brownies and Girl Guides in Book 4 '10 Days in March.. Possibilities' Chapter 8 © 2018 by, Eleanor Deckert published by FreisenPress.

25   Songwriter: Daniel Gaston Ash, Kevin Haskins, David Jay Eclipse lyrics © Universal Music Publishing Group

26   Songwriters: John Denver, Michael C. Taylor, Mike Taylor The Eagle And The Hawk lyrics © Kobalt Music Publishing Ltd., Reservoir Media Management INC

27   Songwriters: Bill Danoff, John Denver, Taffy Nivert Danoff Country Roads lyrics © Warner/Chappell Music, Inc., Reservoir One Music, Kobalt Music Publishing Ltd., Reservoir Media Management INC, BMG Rights Management US, LLC

28   I invented 'Talking Quilts' as an educational 'toy' to encourage language development. Alternating denim and picture squares of fabric all

relating to a theme stimulate story telling, learning, questions and pretend. See photos on author's web page www.eleanordeckert.com '10 Days in April... detour through breast cancer' Chapter 10. by, Eleanor Deckert © 2018 published by FreisenPress.

29 Songwriter: John Denver I Want To Live lyrics © Warner/Chappell Music, Inc., Kobalt Music Publishing Ltd.

Review

A personal memoir about the experience of treatment of breast cancer in a journal style.

A beautiful, touching book; by offering your own vulnerability, you really connect to the reader. Your thoughts and struggles... and journey you were on is very relatable to those who have cancer, the those who know someone with cancer...

It also has an uplifting and touching ending, which... emphasizes your personal growth.

—Evaluation Editor, FriesenPress

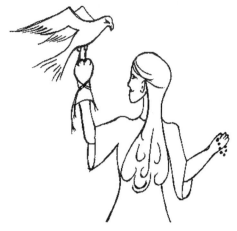

About The Author

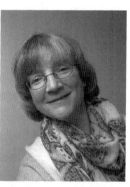

"You can write a book about your experiences!" my well meaning friend suggested. "You can keep a Journal!"

"You'll make lots of friends!" she tried to encourage me.

"You'll help a lot of people!" yet another suggestion.

Not very likely! I don't want to remember any of this... no Journal... no friends... and it will be hard enough to take care of my own Self, I have no intention of listening to or helping anyone else.

That was the attitude I packed up and took with me when I traveled five hours from home to enter the cancer centre for daily radiation treatments.

Dizzy with inner conflict, haunted by fears of technological interventions, confused by conflicting advice, unprepared for scientific interference in my Mother Nature lifestyle, I had never had to reconcile my spiritual beliefs with a traumatic personal decision-making process.

Thankfully, support came in many and varied ways.

I made it through the detour.

Printed in Canada